The Essential
Low FODMAP Diet
Cookbook

150 Easy & Delicious Recipes to Manage IBS and Digestive Disorders.
Includes a Complete 30-Day Meal Plan for Gut Wellness.

Vita Johnston

Copyright © 2024 by Vita Johnston. All rights reserved.

No part of this publication may be reproduced, distributed, or transmitted in any form or by any means, including photocopying, recording, or other electronic or mechanical methods, without the prior written permission of the publisher, except in the case of brief quotations included in critical reviews and specific other noncommercial uses permitted by copyright law.

Disclaimer

The content of this book is for general information purposes only and is not intended as medical advice. The author and publisher are not medical professionals. Before starting any new diet program, it is recommended that you consult with a healthcare provider.

The dietary guidance and recipes in this book are intended as suggestions only and may not be suitable for everyone. It is the reader's responsibility to ensure that any food ingredients or dietary practices are appropriate for their specific health conditions.

The author and publisher disclaim any liability concerning the use of this information, and no warranty is implied beyond what is described in this disclaimer.

Table of Contents

Introduction 8

Chapter 1: Understanding the Low FODMAP Diet 10

   The Science Behind the Diet 10

   Explanation of FODMAPs and Their Impact on the Gut 10

   The Link Between FODMAPs and Gastrointestinal Issues Like IBS 11

   Why Choose the Low FODMAP Diet? Benefits and Challenges 12

   How to Start and Proceed with the Low FODMAP Diet 14

   Practical Tips for Managing the Low FODMAP Diet 16

Chapter 2: Breakfasts 19

   Spanish Tortilla 19

   Golden Polenta Cakes 19

   Vanilla Rice Pudding 20

   Turkey and Cheddar Breakfast Biscuits 20

   Classic Shakshuka 21

   Sweet Potato and Walnuts Bowl 21

   Berries Chia Pudding 22

   Egg Bites with Ham 22

   Quinoa Pancakes 23

   Walnut and Seeds Granola 24

   Low FODMAP French Toast 24

   Classic Polenta 25

   Mediterranean Vegetable Omelet 25

   Blueberry Chia Overnight Oats 26

   Berry Smoothie 26

   Buckwheat Crepes 27

Chapter 3: Starters, Snacks and Soups 28

   Italian Bruschetta 28

   Stuffed Peppers with Quinoa and Turkey 28

   Smoked Salmon Roll-Ups 29

Baked Parmesan Zucchini Fries 29

Lemon Herb Chicken Skewers 30

Prosciutto Wrapped Honeydew Melon 30

Cucumber and Hummus Bites 31

Spicy BBQ Chicken Wings 31

Vegetarian Spring Rolls 32

Balsamic Glazed Meatballs 33

Roasted Chickpeas 33

Miso Soup with Tofu and Greens 34

Carrot Ginger Soup 34

Thai Coconut Chicken Soup 35

Turkey and Rice Soup 35

Minestrone 36

Pumpkin Soup 36

Moroccan Spiced Vegetable Soup 37

Zucchini Cream Soup 37

Vegetable Broth 38

Lentil Soup with Carrots and Kale 38

Seafood Chowder 39

Chapter 4: Salads and Sides **40**

Carrot and Walnut Salad 40

Egg Salad with Dill 40

Quinoa Tabbouleh 41

Arugula and Shaved Parmesan Salad 41

Roasted Potato Salad 42

Zucchini Noodle Salad 42

Rice Salad with Fennel and Orange 43

Mini Caprese Salad 43

Grilled Chicken Caesar Salad 44

Garlic-Infused Olive Oil Sautéed Spinach 44

Pumpkin and Spinach Salad 45

Cucumber and Radish Salad 45

Broccoli and Bacon Salad 46

Stir-Fried Bell Peppers 46

Spinach and Cheese Stuffed Potatoes 47

Sautéed Broccoli with Garlic Oil 47

Butternut Squash Risotto 48

Chicken and Orange Salad 49

Roasted Red Cabbage Steaks 49

Ratatouille 50

Grilled Zucchini Ribbons 50

Lactose-Free Potato Gratin 51

Green Beans with Toasted Almonds 51

Quinoa and Vegetable Stuffed Peppers 52

Chapter 5: Poultry, Meat and Seafood 53

Grilled Chicken with Herbs 53

Rosemary Infused Roast Beef 53

Maple Mustard Pork Chops 54

Lemon Herb Roast Chicken 54

Prosciutto Wrapped Chicken 55

Balsamic Glazed Beef Ribs 56

Turkey Meatballs 57

Lemon Thyme Pork Tenderloin 57

Beef Stir Fry 58

Spiced Moroccan Chicken 58

Maple-Glazed Chicken Breasts 59

Spiced Chicken Drumettes 59

Moroccan Spiced Lamb Ribs 60

Herbed Turkey Burgers 60

Beef and Fennel Casserole 61

Roasted Chicken with Fennel and Carrots 61

Pork Tenderloin with Oregano and Orange 62

Italian Meatloaf 62

Beef Bolognese 63

Grilled Tilapia with Oregano and Olive Oil 63

Spicy Grilled Tuna with Salsa 64

Lemon Pepper Salmon 64

Seafood Paella 65

Cilantro Lime Shrimp 65

Cod in Parsley Sauce 66

Sea Bass with Fennel and Tomatoes 66

Prawn Stir Fry 67

Grilled Scallops with Basil Dressing 67

Grilled Mackerel with Herb Salad 68

Fennel and Salmon Bake 68

Baked Trout with Dill and Lemon 69

Sesame Crusted Tuna Steak 69

Chapter 6: Cakes, Snacks and Desserts 70

Carrot Cake 70

Chocolate Pudding 70

Zucchini and Cheese Scones 71

Peanut Butter Cookies 72

Almond Joy Bars 72

Lemon Cupcakes 73

Pumpkin Pie 73

Oatmeal Raisin Cookies 74

Sesame Rice Cakes 74

Orange Polenta Cake 75

Oat and Peanut Butter Energy Balls 75

Chocolate Cake 76

Coconut Rice Pudding 76

Gluten-Free Pumpkin Bread 77

Cheese Crackers 78

Sweet Potato Brownies 78

Cheddar and Herb Muffins 79

Almond Banana Muffins 79

Baked Oatmeal Cups 80
Chapter 7: Condiments 81
Garlic-Infused Olive Oil 81
Lemon Tahini Dressing 81
Pesto 82
Barbecue Sauce 82
Cucumber Dill Yogurt Dip 83
Green Onion Aioli 83
Italian Dressing 84
Tzatziki Sauce 84
Hummus 85
Cranberry Sauce 85
Mint Yogurt Sauce 86
Vegan Alfredo Sauce 86
Nut Butter 87
Chapter 8: Drinks 88
Herbal Iced Tea 88
Lemon Lime Soda 88
Peppermint Tea 89
Cucumber Mint Infused Water 89
Berry Lemonade 90
Ginger Turmeric Tea 90
Maple Cinnamon Latte 91
Kiwi Strawberry Slush 91
Golden Latte 92
Chapter 9: 30-Day Meal Plan 93
Conclusion 99
Appendix 1: Low FODMAP and High FODMAP Food Lists 101
Appendix 2: Resource Recommendation 104
Appendix 3: Measurement Conversions 105

Introduction

Welcome to your journey towards a happier, healthier gut! If you're reading this, you might be one of the many who struggle daily with the discomfort and challenges of Irritable Bowel Syndrome (IBS). You know all too well the confusion and frustration that comes with this condition, not to mention the often debilitating symptoms that disrupt your day-to-day life. But what if I told you that relief could be as simple as turning the pages of this book?

My own battle with IBS led me down a path filled with countless doctor visits, myriad treatments, and endless dietary advice that seemed to lead nowhere. It was only when I discovered the Low FODMAP Diet that I truly began to reclaim my life and manage my symptoms effectively. Having experienced significant relief from my symptoms, I was inspired to share this success through "The Essential Low FODMAP Diet Cookbook," designed to offer you an easy-to-follow roadmap to gut health and overall well-being.

This book is more than just a collection of recipes. It's a toolkit packed with scientifically backed insights and practical advice that addresses the root of your digestive woes. Every recipe has been tailored to ensure it is low in Fermentable Oligosaccharides, Monosaccharides, Disaccharides, and Polyols, which are the complex terms for the carbohydrates that could be troubling your digestive system.

On this gastronomic adventure, you'll learn the dual power of flavor and nutrition working together to soothe your symptoms. The dishes have been designed to be as delicious as they are healing, dispelling the myth that a therapeutic diet must be bland or restrictive. From hearty breakfasts to satisfying dinners and even delectable desserts, you'll find that each meal brings you one step closer to a more vibrant and symptom-free life.

But this book does more than feed your stomach; it also aims to educate and empower. As we progress to Chapter 1, "Understanding the Low FODMAP Diet", you'll gain a basic understanding of why certain foods can trigger unpleasant symptoms and how your body reacts to different types of food, benefits and challenges of the diet as well as practical tips to manage it smoothly.

This knowledge is power - the power to make knowledgeable choices regarding your diet and to manage your health effectively.

Embark on this transformative journey with me. Let's explore the possibilities that await when you combine the science of nutrition with the art of cooking, all tailored to nurture your body and appease your taste buds. Together, we can turn the page on IBS and start a new chapter in your life—one filled with health, happiness, and delicious food. Join me as we delve into the essentials of the Low FODMAP Diet and discover how you can live well, one meal at a time.

Chapter 1: Understanding the Low FODMAP Diet

The Low FODMAP Diet is a scientifically backed nutritional approach explicitly developed to alleviate symptoms in people struggling with Irritable Bowel Syndrome (IBS) and other functional gastrointestinal disorders. This section of the book delves into the foundational science of the diet, explains what FODMAPs are and how they affect the gut, and discusses their connection to common gastrointestinal issues.

The Science Behind the Diet

The diet originated from research conducted by a team at Monash University in Melbourne, Australia. They discovered that certain types of carbohydrates were not absorbed well in the small intestine and could trigger symptoms in individuals with sensitive guts. The acronym FODMAP stands for Fermentable Oligo-, Di-, Monosaccharides, And Polyols - specific types of short-chain carbohydrates that, when poorly absorbed, ferment in the colon. This fermentation process produces gas, which leads to bloating, pain, and other discomforts associated with IBS.

Explanation of FODMAPs and Their Impact on the Gut

FODMAPs include various sugars and fibers present in many common foods, which can draw excess fluid into the gut and generate gas when fermented by bacteria in the large intestine. Here are some examples of high FODMAP foods in each category:

- **Oligosaccharides:** Included in foods such as rye, wheat, garlic, and onions, these carbohydrates are prevalent in man's diets and are known for causing digestive issues in sensitive individuals.

- **Disaccharides:** Lactose from dairy products, such as milk, yogurt, and soft cheeses, is problematic for individuals who lack the enzyme lactase, which is necessary for its digestion.

- **Monosaccharides:** Fructose, a simple sugar found in high concentrations in apples, honey, and high-fructose corn syrups, can exacerbate symptoms when it is more abundant than glucose in the diet.

- **Polyols:** These sugar alcohols, like sorbitol and mannitol, are found in some fruits and vegetables, including mushrooms and stone fruits, as well as in artificial sweeteners.

When people with IBS or similar gastrointestinal sensitivities consume foods high in FODMAPs, they often experience an increase in symptoms due to the extra gas produced and the water pulled into the gut. This can lead to bloating, pain, diarrhea, and constipation.

The Link Between FODMAPs and Gastrointestinal Issues Like IBS

Research has robustly supported the link between the consumption of high FODMAP foods and the worsening of IBS symptoms. The connection stems from how these carbohydrates affect the balance of the intestinal environment:

1. **Osmotic Effect:** FODMAPs draw water into the intestine, which can alter bowel movements and lead to diarrhea or constipation.

2. **Fermentation and Gas Production:** As FODMAPs are fermented by gut bacteria, they produce gases, that can lead to significant bloating, cramping, and discomfort.

Many clinical studies have shown that individuals with IBS who try a Low FODMAP Diet face a significant reduction in these symptoms. In these studies, around 70% of participants reported improvement, making this diet one of the most effective nutritional therapies for managing IBS.

By understanding the types of foods that are high in FODMAPs and learning how to limit them, people can effectively manage and often significantly reduce their gastrointestinal symptoms. The Low FODMAP Diet is not about eliminating these foods forever but about understanding personal thresholds and managing intake to maintain a balanced, symptom-free life.

Why Choose the Low FODMAP Diet? Benefits and Challenges

Adopting a new diet can be a significant decision, especially with the promise of alleviating chronic symptoms. The Low FODMAP Diet is increasingly recommended for people with IBS and other similar digestive disorders. However, the diet also presents challenges.

Benefits of the Low FODMAP Diet

Symptom Relief

The most compelling reason to choose the Low FODMAP Diet is the effective relief of symptoms. Numerous studies have shown that reducing the intake of FODMAPs can dramatically alleviate common symptoms of IBS, including:

- **Bloating:** Reducing FODMAP intake can decrease gas production and bloating.

- **Abdominal Pain:** Many report a significant reduction in the severity and frequency of abdominal pain.

- **Diarrhea and Constipation:** By stabilizing digestion, the diet helps normalize bowel movements.

Patients often experience improvement within just a few weeks of starting the diet, providing a quicker sense of relief compared to some other treatment strategies.

Improved Overall Well-being

Beyond digestive symptoms, many individuals find that managing their diet helps improve overall energy levels, mental clarity, and emotional health. The reduction in pain and discomfort contributes to better sleep and reduced anxiety related to digestive issues.

Empowerment and Control

Living with digestive disorders can often make individuals feel powerless over their health. The Low FODMAP Diet empowers you with the knowledge to identify which foods trigger your symptoms, allowing you to make informed decisions about your diet. This knowledge grants a sense of control over your health and well-being.

Challenges of the Low FODMAP Diet

While the benefits of the Low FODMAP Diet are significant, the path is not without its hurdles. Understanding these challenges can prepare you for a more successful dietary transition.

Diet Complexity and Restrictiveness

The diet begins with an elimination phase, where all high FODMAP foods are removed. This phase can be quite restrictive and complex, as it requires a thorough understanding of which foods contain high levels of FODMAPs. Overwhelming feelings may result from this, especially at the start.

Social and Lifestyle Adjustments

Dietary restrictions can affect social interactions, such as going to events where food is served or dining out. Finding suitable food options that adhere to the low FODMAP guidelines can be challenging, potentially leading to feelings of isolation or exclusion.

Initial Increase in Symptoms

Some individuals may experience an initial increase in symptoms as their body adjusts to the new diet. This can be discouraging, but it is typically temporary as the gut flora adapts to the changes in diet.

Maintaining Nutritional Balance

Ensuring a balanced and nutritionally adequate diet while adhering to the Low FODMAP Diet might be quite a challenge. The elimination of certain fruits, vegetables, and grains can potentially lead to deficiencies if not carefully managed.

Choosing the Low FODMAP Diet involves weighing these benefits and challenges against your personal health goals and lifestyle. By doing so, you can embark on this dietary journey well-prepared and supported, enhancing your opportunities to better life quality by alleviating symptoms.

How to Start and Proceed with the Low FODMAP Diet

Embarking on the Low FODMAP Diet is a transformative journey that can significantly improve gastrointestinal health, particularly for those suffering from IBS and related digestive disorders. This subchapter provides a step-by-step guide on how to start and maintain this diet, emphasizing the crucial role of portion control in managing FODMAP intake.

Starting the Low FODMAP Diet

Step 1: Preparation and Planning

Before beginning the Low FODMAP Diet, it's important to arm yourself with knowledge and prepare your kitchen. This preparation includes:

- **Educating Yourself:** Arm yourself with knowledge about the diet. Learn about the foods that are high and low in FODMAPs. Use various resources to understand food alternatives and meal planning (Appendix 2).

- **Consulting a Healthcare Professional:** Ideally, a dietitian experienced in the Low FODMAP Diet can assist you in navigating the process, ensuring you maintain a balanced diet while following the restrictions.

- **Purging and Restocking:** Clear out high FODMAP foods from your pantry and refrigerator, and restock with Low FODMAP alternatives.

Step 2: Elimination Phase

- **Strict Avoidance:** Eliminate all high FODMAP foods from your diet. This stage typically lasts 4 to 6 weeks and is crucial for resetting your system.

- **Monitoring Symptoms:** Keep a detailed food and symptom diary to record your meals and any resulting symptoms you experience. This record will be invaluable for identifying which foods you can tolerate in later phases.

Step 3: Reintroduction Phase

Gradual Reintroduction: Slowly reintroduce high FODMAP foods one at a time, in a controlled manner, to identify which specific FODMAPs trigger symptoms. Usually, it becomes obvious within 24-48 hours. This phase can take several weeks as you test each FODMAP group methodically.

- **Assessing Tolerance:** Continue to use your food and symptom diary to record reactions to each reintroduced food, noting the severity and type of symptoms experienced.

Step 4: Personalization Phase

- **Customizing Your Diet:** Based on the findings from the reintroduction phase, you can begin to personalize your diet to include as many foods as possible while managing symptoms.

- **Long-term Management:** The final diet should be less restrictive but still mindful of your identified triggers, aiming for the broadest possible variety of foods to ensure nutritional balance.

Practical Tips for Managing the Low FODMAP Diet

Successfully managing the Low FODMAP Diet involves more than understanding what to eat - it's about adjusting to a new lifestyle. This subchapter provides practical advice on how to emotionally and practically adapt to the diet.

Adjusting Emotionally

- **Stay Positive:** Focus on the benefits you'll gain from managing your symptoms rather than the foods you avoid.
- **Seek Support:** Connect with online forums, local support groups, or counseling if you find the diet change overwhelming. Search for "Low FODMAP" in groups on platforms like Facebook. These groups can provide support, share experiences, tips and coping strategies, exchange recipes.
- **Educate Others:** Inform your family and friends about your dietary needs to make social gatherings easier. The more they understand, the more they can support you.

Dealing with Cravings

Find Substitutes: Look for low FODMAP alternatives to satisfy your cravings. Explore Low FODMAP recipes using gluten-free grains or lactose-free products to mimic traditional flavors and textures. If you love garlic, for instance, try garlic-infused oil that is low FODMAP.

Shopping Tips

- **Read Labels:** Always check food labels for high FODMAP ingredients. Ingredients are always listed by quantity, from highest to lowest. Opt for gluten-free options and familiarize yourself with brands that offer Low FODMAP certified products.
- **Shop the Perimeter:** Most fresh fruits, vegetables, and proteins low in FODMAPs are located around the store's perimeter. Processed foods in the middle aisles often contain high FODMAP ingredients.

- **Use a Shopping List:** Keep a list of "safe" low FODMAP foods on your phone or in your wallet, which you can refer to while shopping.

Stocking Your Pantry

- **Plan Ahead:** Meal planning is crucial. Plan your meals for the week to avoid last-minute decisions that might not be FODMAP-friendly.

- **Essentials List:** Create a list of low FODMAP pantry essentials such as gluten-free pasta, rice, canned vegetables with no added onion or garlic, and herbal teas.

- **Organize Your Space:** Dedicate an area of your pantry and refrigerator to low FODMAP foods to avoid confusion with other family members' foods.

- **Batch Cooking:** Prepare and freeze low FODMAP meals for busy days. This prevents the temptation to eat something high in FODMAPs.

Dining Out and Traveling

- **Restaurant Research:** Before dining out, research restaurants and menus online to find those with low FODMAP options. Don't hesitate to call ahead and discuss your dietary needs with the chef.

- **Be Specific:** When ordering, be specific about your dietary needs. For example, ask for no onion or garlic and request dressings and sauces on the side.

- **Travel Prepared:** When traveling, pack low FODMAP snacks like homemade trail mix, rice cakes, and lactose-free yogurt. Check for grocery stores near your accommodation where you can stock up on essentials.

Adjusting to Life on the Low FODMAP Diet

Embracing the Low FODMAP Diet fully often requires significant changes to your daily habits, but with the right tools, resources and mindset, these changes can become a seamless part of your lifestyle. By applying these useful suggestions, you can uphold your diet with confidence and continue to enjoy a full and active life, free from the discomfort of IBS symptoms.

Chapter 2: Breakfasts
Spanish Tortilla

Prep. time: 10 min **Total time:** 30 min **Servings:** 4

Ingredients:

- 8 eggs
- 1 cup diced potatoes (boiled until just tender)
- 1/2 cup finely chopped green onions (only the green parts)
- 1/4 cup chopped fresh parsley
- 1/4 cup olive oil
- Salt and pepper to taste

Nutrition (per serving):

320 calories | 22g fat | 18g carbs | 14g protein | 3g sugar

Directions:

1. Whisk the eggs, parsley, salt, and pepper together in a large mixing bowl until well combined.
2. Add olive oil to a non-stick skillet and warm to medium. Add the boiled potatoes and green onions, and sauté for about 5 minutes until they start to get a golden color.
3. Pour the egg blend over the potatoes and onions in the pan. Cook over low heat without stirring for about 10–15 minutes until the eggs are just set and the bottom is golden.
4. Place a large plate over the frying pan and gently turn the tortilla onto the plate, then ease it back into the skillet to cook the other side for another 5 minutes.
5. Transfer the tortilla to a plate and allow to cool slightly before cutting it into wedges.

Golden Polenta Cakes

Prep. time: 15 min **Total time:** 40 min **Servings:** 4

Ingredients:

- 1 cup instant polenta
- 4 cups water
- 1 teaspoon salt
- 1 cup chopped spinach (fresh or frozen and thawed)
- 1/2 cup grated Parmesan cheese
- 2 tablespoons olive oil

Nutrition (per serving):

290 calories | 10g fat | 40g carbs | 9g protein | 1g sugar

Directions:

1. In a medium saucepan, boil water and salt. Gradually whisk in the polenta. Next, reduce the heat to the minimum temperature and stir continuously until the polenta is thick and soft, which should take about 5-7 minutes.
2. Remove from heat and mix with the chopped spinach and grated Parmesan cheese until well combined.
3. Spread the polenta mixture into a greased rectangular dish or tray. Smooth the top and let it cool until set about 15 minutes.
4. Once set, cut the polenta into squares or circles using a cookie cutter.
5. Add the olive oil to a skillet and heat it to medium.
6. Fry the polenta cakes until golden and crispy on both sides, about 4 minutes per side. Serve warm.

Vanilla Rice Pudding

Prep. time: 5 min   **Total time:** 40 min   **Servings:** 4

Ingredients:

- 1/2 cup uncooked white rice
- 3 cups lactose-free milk
- 1/4 cup granulated sugar
- 1 vanilla bean, cut lengthwise in half, with the seeds removed
- 1 cinnamon stick
- Pinch of salt

Nutrition (per serving):

220 calories | 2.5g fat | 44g carbs | 5g protein | 20g sugar

Directions:

1. In a medium saucepan, combine the rice, lactose-free milk, sugar, vanilla bean (including the pod), cinnamon stick, and a pinch of salt.
2. Heat the mixture on medium-high. After bringing it to a boil, bring the heat down and let it simmer. Stir often to keep the rice from adhering to the bottom of the pan.
3. Allow to cook for around 30 to 35 minutes, until the rice is tender and the mixture has a creamy texture.
4. Take the pan off the heat, and remove and discard the vanilla bean pod and cinnamon stick.
5. Spoon the pudding into serving bowls. You can serve it warm or cool it in the refrigerator if you prefer it chilled. For more sweetness, add a bit of maple syrup on top.

Turkey and Cheddar Breakfast Biscuits

Prep. time: 15 min   **Total time:** 35 min   **Servings:** 4

Ingredients:

- 2 cups gluten-free biscuit mix
- 2/3 cup lactose-free milk
- 1/4 cup cold, cubed, unsalted butter
- 8 slices turkey breast
- 4 slices aged cheddar cheese
- 1 egg, beaten)

Nutrition (per serving):

360 calories | 18g fat | 34g carbs | 18g protein | 2g sugar

Directions:

1. Heat your oven to 425°F (220°C) and prepare a baking sheet.
2. In a large bowl, combine the gluten-free biscuit mix with the cold, cubed butter. To make the mixture resemble coarse crumbs, add the butter into the mixture using your fingers or a pastry blender.
3. Gradually stir in the lactose-free milk until the dough comes together. Be careful not to overmix.
4. Set the dough on a lightly floured surface (use gluten-free flour) and knead gently 4-5 times. Roll it out to a thickness of roughly one inch, and use a biscuit cutter to cut out rounds.
5. Set the biscuits on the lined baking sheet. Apply beaten egg to the tops for a golden sheen. Bake up to 15 minutes, or until golden brown, in a preheated oven.
6. Once baked, split the biscuits while still warm and fill each with a slice of turkey and cheddar. Serve immediately.

Classic Shakshuka

Prep. time: 10 min **Total time:** 30 min **Servings:** 4

Ingredients:

- 1 tablespoon garlic-infused olive oil
- 1 large red bell pepper, diced
- 1 (14-ounce) can of diced tomatoes (no onion or garlic)
- 1/2 cup tomato passata (ensure no garlic or onion is added)
- 1 teaspoon cumin
- 1 teaspoon smoked paprika
- 1/4 teaspoon cayenne pepper (optional, adjust to taste)
- Salt and pepper, to taste
- 4-6 large eggs
- 1/4 cup chopped fresh onion greens
- Fresh cilantro or parsley for garnish (optional)

Directions:

1. Warm garlic-infused olive oil in a sizeable skillet over medium heat. Add diced red bell pepper; sauté for 5 minutes.
2. Stir in diced tomatoes, tomato passata, cumin, smoked paprika, and cayenne pepper. Season with salt and pepper. Simmer for 10 minutes.
3. Create wells in the sauce, and break an egg into each one. Cover and cook for 5-7 minutes until the eggs are set.
4. Garnish with green onion tops and cilantro or parsley.

Nutrition (per serving):

180 calories | 10g fat | 13g carbs | 12g protein | 8g sugar

Sweet Potato and Walnuts Bowl

Prep. time: 15 min **Total time:** 35 min **Servings:** 2

Ingredients:

- 1 large sweet potato, peeled and diced
- 1 tablespoon olive oil
- 1/4 teaspoon salt
- 1/4 teaspoon black pepper
- 1/2 cup chopped walnuts
- 2 tablespoons pumpkin seeds
- 2 tablespoons chia seeds
- 1/2 cup lactose-free plain yogurt
- 1/4 teaspoon cinnamon
- 1 tablespoon maple syrup (optional)

Directions:

1. Heat the oven to 400°F (200°C).
2. Mix the diced sweet potato with olive oil, salt, and pepper on a baking sheet. Spread in a single layer.
3. Roast in the oven, once preheated, for 20 minutes or until tender and lightly browned.
4. While the sweet potatoes are roasting, toast the walnuts and pumpkin seeds in a dry skillet over medium heat for 5 minutes, stirring regularly to avoid burning.
5. After taking the sweet potatoes out of the oven, let them cool a little.
6. Combine the roasted sweet potato, toasted nuts and seeds, chia seeds, lactose-free yogurt, and cinnamon. Stir gently to combine. Drizzle with maple syrup if desired.
7. Serve warm.

Berries Chia Pudding

Prep. time: 5 min **Total time:** 5 min **Servings:** 2

Ingredients:

- 1/4 cup chia seeds
- 1 cup coconut milk or other Low FODMAP milk (unsweetened)
- 1/2 teaspoon vanilla extract
- 1 tablespoon maple syrup (optional for sweetness)
- Fresh strawberries, raspberries or blueberries for topping
- A pinch of cinnamon (optional for flavor)

Directions:

1. Chia seeds, almond milk, vanilla extract, and maple syrup, if using, should all be combined in a bowl. Toss to blend well.
2. After letting the mixture settle for roughly ten minutes, give it another toss to loosen up any chia seed clusters.
3. Once the mixture thickens and takes on the consistency of pudding, cover the bowl and refrigerate for at least two hours or overnight.
4. Serve the chia pudding chilled, topped with fresh berries and a sprinkle of cinnamon if desired.

Nutrition (per serving):

167 calories | 9.75g fat | 20g carbs | 3g protein | 8g sugar

Egg Bites with Ham

Prep. time: 10 min **Total time:** 30 min **Servings:** 4

Ingredients:

- 6 large eggs
- 1/4 cup lactose-free milk
- 1/4 teaspoon salt
- 1/4 teaspoon black pepper
- 1/2 cup grated cheddar cheese (lactose-free if necessary)
- 1/2 cup diced ham
- 1/4 cup chopped spinach

Nutrition (per serving):

230 calories | 16g fat | 2g carbs | 20g protein | 1g sugar

Directions:

1. Set the oven temperature to 350°F (175°C). Prepare silicone muffin cups on a baking tray or grease a muffin pan.
2. Mix the eggs, lactose-free milk, pepper, and salt thoroughly in a sizable mixing dish.
3. Add the chopped spinach, diced ham, and shredded cheddar cheese.
4. Spoon the egg mixture into each prepared muffin cups, filling them about two thirds of the way to the top.
5. Bake for 20 minutes in a preheated oven or until the egg bites' tops are gently brown and set. Take them out of the oven, then allow to cool down for a few minutes before taking out of the muffin tray.
6. Serve warm.

Quinoa Pancakes

Prep. time: 10 min   **Total time:** 25 min   **Servings:** 4

Ingredients:

- 1/2 cup raw white quinoa
- 1 cup water (for soaking)
- 1/2 cup water or almond milk (for blending)
- 2 tsp vegetable oil plus more for cooking
- 1 large egg
- 1 teaspoon baking powder
- 1/2 teaspoon salt
- Optional toppings: maple syrup (in small quantities), fresh berries, or lactose-free yogurt

Nutrition (per serving):

210 calories | 10g fat | 24g carbs | 6g protein | 1g sugar

Directions:

1. Put the quinoa in a bowl and add one cup of water to cover it. Let soak overnight in the refrigerator.
2. Drain and rinse the soaked quinoa thoroughly.
3. In a blender, combine the soaked quinoa, 1/2 cup of water or almond milk, vegetable oil, and egg. Blend until the mixture is smooth.
4. Transfer into a bowl and mix in the salt and baking powder.
5. Lightly oil and heat a skillet over medium heat.
6. For each pancake, transfer 1/4 cup of batter to the skillet. Cook for two to three minutes on each side or until the edges are dry and bubbles start to appear.
7. Bake for a further two to three minutes or until golden brown.
8. Serve hot with toppings such as lactose-free yogurt, fresh berries and maple syrup.

Walnut and Seeds Granola

Prep. time: 10 min **Total time:** 30 min **Servings:** 6

Ingredients:

- 2 cups rolled oats (gluten-free if necessary)
- 1 cup chopped walnuts
- 1/2 cup pumpkin seeds
- 1/4 cup sunflower seeds
- 1/4 cup maple syrup
- 1/4 cup coconut oil, melted
- 1 teaspoon vanilla extract
- 1/2 teaspoon cinnamon
- 1/4 teaspoon salt

Nutrition (per serving):

345 calories | 27g fat | 23g carbs | 8g protein | 7g sugar

Directions:

1. Preheat oven to 300°F (150°C)
2. Combine the oats, walnuts, pumpkin seeds, and sunflower seeds in a sizable mixing dish.
3. Combine the maple syrup, melted coconut oil, salt, cinnamon and vanilla extract in another bowl.
4. Stir together the oat mixture and wet ingredients until well-coated.
5. Evenly distribute the mixture onto a baking sheet covered with parchment paper.
6. Bake for 20 minutes in an oven, tossing once to achieve even baking.
7. Take out of the oven and allow to cool completely on the baking sheet.
8. Keep in an airtight container at room temperature.

Low FODMAP French Toast

Prep. time: 10 min **Total time:** 20 min **Servings:** 4

Ingredients:

- 8 slices gluten-free bread
- 4 eggs
- 1 cup lactose-free milk
- 1 teaspoon vanilla extract
- 1/2 teaspoon cinnamon
- 2 tablespoons maple syrup (for serving)
- Butter or non-dairy alternative (for frying)

Nutrition (per serving):

280 calories | 11g fat | 36g carbs | 11g protein | 12g sugar

Directions:

1. Whisk together the eggs with lactose-free milk, vanilla extract, and cinnamon in a bowl.
2. Add a little quantity of butter or a non-dairy alternative to a big skillet or griddle and heat it over medium heat.
3. Dip each slice of gluten-free bread in the egg mixture, letting it soak for a few seconds on each side.
4. Cook the soaked bread slices on the hot pan for about 2-3 minutes on each side or until each side is golden brown.
5. Serve the French toast hot, drizzled with maple syrup.

Classic Polenta

Prep. time: 5 min **Total time:** 35 min **Servings:** 4

Ingredients:

- 1 cup polenta (coarse cornmeal)
- 4 cups water
- 1 teaspoon salt
- 2 tablespoons butter (lactose-free if necessary)
- 1/4 cup grated Parmesan cheese
- Fresh herbs for garnish (such as parsley or thyme)

Directions:

1. Heat the water and salt in a big pot until they start to boil.
2. Gradually whisk in the polenta to prevent clumping.
3. Reduce heat to low and, stirring constantly, continue cooking the polenta until it thickens and becomes creamy, about 25-30 minutes.
4. Take off the heat and add the butter and grated Parmesan cheese until well combined.
5. Serve hot, garnished with fresh herbs.

Nutrition (per serving):

250 calories | 9g fat | 34g carbs | 6g protein | 1g sugar

Mediterranean Vegetable Omelet

Prep. time: 5 min **Total time:** 15 min **Servings:** 2

Ingredients:

- 1 cup rolled oats
- 2 cup unsweetened almond milk
- 1 medium banana, mashed
- 1/2 teaspoon vanilla extract
- 1/2 teaspoon ground cinnamon
- pinch of salt

Nutrition (per serving):

320 calories | 23g fat | 8g carbs | 21g protein | 3g sugar

Directions:

1. In a bowl, whisk together the eggs, lactose-free milk, salt, and pepper.
2. Heat the garlic-infused olive oil in a non-stick skillet over medium heat.
3. Swirl the egg mixture into the skillet to coat the bottom evenly.
4. As the eggs start to firm up, carefully lift the edges with a spatula, permitting the uncooked egg to flow beneath.
5. When the omelet is mostly set but still slightly runny on top, sprinkle diced tomatoes, bell peppers, black olives, and crumbled feta cheese over half of the omelet.
6. Flip the other half of the omelet over the filling.
7. Cook for another 2 minutes, then slide onto a plate.
8. Garnish with fresh basil or parsley. Serve hot.

Blueberry Chia Overnight Oats

Prep. time: 5 min   **Total time:** 8 hr 5 min   **Servings:** 2

Ingredients:

- 1 cup rolled oats (gluten-free if necessary)
- 1 cup lactose-free milk or almond milk
- 1/2 cup fresh blueberries
- 2 tablespoons chia seeds
- 2 tablespoons maple syrup
- 1/2 teaspoon vanilla extract
- A pinch of salt

Nutrition (per serving):

350 calories | 9g fat | 59g carbs | 10g protein | 18g sugar

Directions:

1. Combine the rolled oats, lactose-free milk, blueberries, chia seeds, a pinch of salt, maple syrup and vanilla extract in a mixing bowl. Stir well to mix.
2. Evenly distribute the mixture between two jars or containers with lids.
3. Seal the containers and place them in the refrigerator overnight, or for at least 8 hours, to let the flavors meld and the oats soften.
4. In the morning, give the oats a good stir. You can add a small amount of lactose-free milk to reach the desired consistency in case the mixture is too thick.
5. Serve cold straight from the refrigerator or let it sit at room temperature for a few minutes. Top with additional fresh blueberries if desired.

Berry Smoothie

Prep. time: 5 min   **Total time:** 5 min   **Servings:** 3

Ingredients:

- 1 cup frozen strawberries
- 1/2 cup frozen blueberries
- 1 medium banana, sliced
- 1 cup lactose-free yogurt or coconut yogurt
- 1/2 cup almond milk
- 1 tablespoon chia seeds
- 1 tablespoon maple syrup (optional, adjust to taste)

Directions:

1. Place the frozen strawberries, blueberries, banana, chia seeds, lactose-free yogurt, almond milk, and maple syrup (if using) in a blender.
2. Blend on high until smooth and creamy. You can add a small amount of additional almond milk to the smoothie, if it's too thick to your liking.
3. If necessary, adjust the sweetness by adding a bit of maple syrup and serve the smoothie immediately

Nutrition (per serving):

280 calories | 8g fat | 46g carbs | 8g protein | 22g sugar

Buckwheat Crepes

Prep. time: 10 min   **Total time:** 30 min   **Servings:** 4

Ingredients:

- 1 cup buckwheat flour
- 1 1/2 cups lactose-free milk or almond milk
- 2 large eggs
- 1/4 teaspoon salt
- 2 tablespoons of melted coconut oil, plus extra for cooking
- 1/2 teaspoon vanilla extract (optional, for sweet crepes)

Nutrition (per serving):

280 calories | 14g fat | 32g carbs | 10g protein | 5g sugar

Directions:

1. In a blender, combine the buckwheat flour, lactose-free milk, eggs, salt, melted coconut oil, and vanilla extract (if making sweet crepes). Blend the batter until it's lump-free and smooth. To make a soft crepe, let the batter sit at room temperature for at least thirty minutes so the flour can absorb the liquid.

2. Preheat a crepe pan or a non-stick skillet over medium heat. Brush the pan lightly with coconut oil.

3. Pour 1/4 cup of the batter into the center of the pan. Then, quickly swirling the crepe pan, spread the batter thinly across the bottom.

4. Cook for 1-2 minutes, or until the edges of the crepe start to lightly brown and lift from the pan. Use a spatula to turn the crepe over and cook the other side for a minute or until lightly golden.

5. Transfer the cooked crepe to a plate. To keep it warm, cover it with a kitchen towel. Continue cooking the remaining batter, adding more coconut oil to the pan as needed.

6. Serve the crepes warm with your choice of low FODMAP fillings, such as strawberries, lactose-free yogurt, a drizzle of maple syrup for sweet crepes, or spinach and shredded cheese for savory crepes.

Chapter 3: Starters, Snacks and Soups
Italian Bruschetta

Prep. time: 10 min   **Total time:** 15 min   **Servings:** 4

Ingredients:

- 1 baguette, sliced into 1/2-inch pieces
- 1/4 cup garlic-infused olive oil
- 2 medium tomatoes, finely chopped
- 8 basil leaves, chopped
- Salt and pepper to taste

Directions:

1. Preheat your oven to 375°F (190°C).
2. Brush each baguette slice lightly with garlic-infused olive oil and then move to a baking sheet.
3. Toast in the oven for roughly five minutes or until the edges are crisp and golden.
4. While the bread is toasting, combine the chopped tomatoes and basil in a small bowl. Season with salt and pepper.
5. Transfer the tomato mixture over the slices of toast just before serving to keep them crispy.

Nutrition (per serving):

200 calories | 10g fat | 24g carbs | 4g protein | 3g sugar

Stuffed Peppers with Quinoa and Turkey

Prep. time: 15 min   **Total time:** 45 min   **Servings:** 4

Ingredients:

- 4 bell peppers with the tops chopped off and the seeds removed
- 1 cup cooked quinoa
- 1/2 pound ground turkey
- 1/4 cup finely chopped green parts of onions
- 1 medium carrot, grated
- 1/2 cup diced tomatoes (canned, no added sugar or garlic)
- 1/4 cup chopped fresh parsley
- 1 tablespoon garlic-infused olive oil
- 1 teaspoon dried oregano
- Salt and pepper to taste

Directions:

1. Preheat your oven to 375°F (190°C).
2. In a skillet, heat the garlic-infused olive oil over medium heat. Then cook ground turkey until browned.
3. Stir in the green onions, grated carrot, and tomatoes, cooking for a few minutes until the vegetables are soft.
4. Take off the heat and add the cooked quinoa, parsley, oregano, salt, and pepper.
5. Stuff the mixture evenly into the hollowed-out bell peppers.
6. Place the stuffed peppers standing up in a baking dish.
7. Place in the oven and bake for around 30 minutes or until the peppers are soft and the filling is hot.

Nutrition (per serving):

250 calories | 10g fat | 27g carbs | 15g protein | 6g sugar

Smoked Salmon Roll-Ups

Prep. time: 10 min   **Total time:** 10 min   **Servings:** 4

Ingredients:

- 8 oz smoked salmon, thinly sliced
- 1/2 cup whipped cream cheese (lactose-free)
- 1/4 cup chopped fresh chives
- 1/4 cup chopped fresh dill
- 1 cucumber, sliced into thin strips
- 1 tablespoon lemon juice
- Pepper to taste

Directions:

1. Combine the whipped cream cheese and chives, lemon juice, pepper, and dill in a small bowl until well combined.
2. Arrange the smoked salmon slices on a flat surface.
3. Apply the cream cheese mixture in a thin layer over each slice of salmon.
4. Place a few strips of cucumber on the edge of each salmon slice.
5. Carefully roll up the salmon tightly around the cucumber.
6. Before serving, let it cool for about half an hour in the refrigerator to help the roll-ups hold their shape.
7. Slice each roll into bite-sized pieces if desired.

Nutrition (per serving):

180 calories | 12g fat | 3g carbs | 15g protein | 1g sugar

Baked Parmesan Zucchini Fries

Prep. time: 10 min   **Total time:** 30 min   **Servings:** 4

Ingredients:

- 4 medium zucchinis, cut into 3-inch sticks
- 1/2 cup grated Parmesan cheese
- 1 cup gluten-free breadcrumbs
- 1 teaspoon garlic-infused olive oil
- 1 teaspoon dried oregano
- 1 teaspoon dried basil
- Salt and pepper to taste
- 1 egg, beaten

Nutrition (per serving):

180 calories | 8g fat | 20g carbs | 8g protein | 5g sugar

Directions:

1. Preheat your oven to 425°F (220°C). Line a baking sheet with parchment paper.
2. In a shallow dish, combine together the grated Parmesan cheese, gluten-free breadcrumbs, oregano, basil, salt, and pepper.
3. Beat the egg with the olive oil scented with garlic in a separate shallow dish.
4. Once each zucchini stick has been thoroughly coated, dip it in the egg mixture and then roll it in the breadcrumb mixture.
5. Place the coated zucchini fries on the prepared baking sheet in a single layer.
6. Bake for about 20 minutes or until golden and crispy in a preheated oven, turning halfway through.

Lemon Herb Chicken Skewers

Prep. time: 15 min **Total time:** 25 min **Servings:** 4

Ingredients:

- 1 1/2 pounds of chicken breast, cut into 1-inch pieces
- 1/4 cup olive oil
- 1/4 cup lemon juice
- 1 tablespoon garlic-infused olive oil
- 1 teaspoon dried oregano
- 1 teaspoon dried thyme
- 1 teaspoon dried rosemary
- Salt and pepper to taste
- Lemon wedges for serving

Directions:

1. In a large bowl, whisk together garlic-infused olive oil, lemon juice, olive oil, oregano, thyme, rosemary, salt, and pepper.
2. Toss the chicken cubes in the marinade to ensure an even coating. For the best flavor, let it sit covered and chilled for at least one hour or overnight.
3. Turn the heat up to medium-high on a grill or grill pan.
4. Thread the marinated chicken cubes onto skewers.
5. Grill the skewers, rotating them occasionally, until the chicken is thoroughly cooked and has clear grill marks, approximately 10 minutes.
6. Serve hot with wedges of lemon on the side.

Nutrition (per serving):

290 calories | 15g fat | 1g carbs | 35g protein | 0g sugar

Prosciutto Wrapped Honeydew Melon

Prep. time: 10 min **Total time:** 10 min **Servings:** 4

Ingredients:

- 1 medium honeydew melon, peeled, seeded, and cut into 16 wedges
- 16 slices of prosciutto, thinly sliced
- Fresh mint leaves, for garnish (optional)

Nutrition (per serving):

150 calories | 5g fat | 15g carbs | 10g protein | 14g sugar

Directions:

1. Wrap each wedge of honeydew melon with a slice of prosciutto, covering the melon slice partially or fully, depending on your preference.
2. Arrange the wrapped melon slices on a platter.
3. Garnish with fresh mint leaves if desired, adding a cool contrast to the sweet and savory flavors.
4. Serve right away or keep chilled in the fridge until you're ready to serve. This dish is best enjoyed chilled.

Cucumber and Hummus Bites

Ingredients:

- 2 large cucumbers, sliced into 1/2-inch thick rounds
- 1 cup low FODMAP hummus (made with canned chickpeas, drained and rinsed, garlic-free)
- 1/4 cup of finely cut red bell pepper
- 1/4 cup carrot, finely grated
- Fresh parsley, chopped

Nutrition (per serving):

90 calories | 5g fat | 10g carbs | 4g protein | 2g sugar

Prep. time: 10 min   **Total time:** 10 min   **Servings:** 4

Directions:

1. Slice the cucumbers into rounds and arrange them on a serving platter.
2. Spoon or pipe about a tablespoon of low-fat hummus onto each cucumber round.
3. Top each hummus dollop with a sprinkle of chopped red bell pepper and grated carrot.
4. Garnish each cucumber bite with a small pinch of chopped fresh parsley.
5. The dish can be served right away or chilled until needed.

Spicy BBQ Chicken Wings

Ingredients:

- 2 pounds chicken wings, tips removed and split at the joint
- 1 tablespoon olive oil
- 1 teaspoon salt
- 1/2 teaspoon black pepper
- 1 cup low FODMAP BBQ sauce (store-bought or homemade)
- 1 tablespoon hot sauce (optional, adjust to taste)
- 1 teaspoon smoked paprika

Nutrition (per serving):

310 calories | 18g fat | 12g carbs | 22g protein | 6g sugar

Prep. time: 10 min   **Total time:** 50 min   **Servings:** 4

Directions:

1. Preheat your oven to 400°F (200°C).
2. Coat the chicken wings thoroughly in a mixture of salt, olive oil and pepper in a big bowl.
3. Place the wings in a single layer on a silicone baking mat or parchment paper-lined baking sheet.
4. Bake the wings for 20 minutes in a preheated oven, then turn them over and bake for another 20 minutes or until crispy and cooked through.
5. While the wings are baking, combine the BBQ sauce, hot sauce, and smoked paprika in a small bowl.
6. After the wings are done, take them out of the oven and toss them in the spicy BBQ sauce mixture until evenly coated.
7. To set the sauce, return the coated wings to the oven and bake for another 10 minutes.
8. Serve hot, garnished with extra hot sauce or fresh herbs.

Vegetarian Spring Rolls

Prep. time: 25 min　　**Total time:** 25 min　　**Servings:** 4

Ingredients:

- 8 rice paper wrappers
- 1 cup thinly sliced red bell pepper
- 1 cup thinly sliced carrots
- 1 cup thinly sliced cucumber
- 1 cup shredded purple cabbage
- 1/2 cup fresh mint leaves
- 1/2 cup fresh basil leaves
- 1/2 cup fresh cilantro
- 1/4 cup hoisin sauce (ensure it's gluten-free and low FODMAP)
- 2 tablespoons peanut butter (optional, for dipping sauce)
- 1 tablespoon soy sauce (for a gluten-free option, use tamari instead)

Directions:

1. Pour warm water into a big bowl. Put a rice paper wrapper into the water. for about 20-30 seconds until it is just soft.
2. Lay the wrapper evenly on a clean work surface. Arrange a few pieces of red bell pepper, carrots, cucumber, and purple cabbage over the lower third of the wrapper, giving each side a space of roughly 1 inch.
3. Top with a few mint, basil, and cilantro leaves.
4. Tightly fold the wrapper's bottom over the filling, then continue rolling after folding in the sides until the seam is sealed.
5. Repeat with the remaining wrappers and fillings.
6. For the dipping sauce, mix soy sauce, peanut butter, and hoisin sauce until smooth iin a small bowl. Adjust consistency with a bit of water if needed.
7. Serve the spring rolls fresh with the dipping sauce on the side.

Nutrition (per serving):

200 calories | 3g fat | 40g carbs | 4g protein | 7g sugar

Balsamic Glazed Meatballs

Ingredients:

- 1 pound of ground beef
- 1/4 cup gluten-free breadcrumbs
- 1/4 cup grated Parmesan cheese
- 1 large egg
- 1 teaspoon dried basil
- 1 teaspoon dried oregano
- Salt and pepper to taste
- 1/2 cup balsamic vinegar
- 2 tablespoons brown sugar
- 1 tablespoon olive oil

Nutrition (per serving):

330 calories | 18g fat | 14g carbs | 26g protein | 8g sugar

Prep. time: 15 min **Total time:** 40 **Servings:** 4

Directions:

1. Preheat your oven to 400°F (200°C). Line a baking sheet with parchment paper.
2. In a large bowl, combine the ground beef, breadcrumbs, Parmesan, egg, basil, oregano, salt, and pepper. Mix well until everything is evenly distributed.
3. Form 1-inch meatballs and place them on the baking sheet.
4. Bake the meatballs for about 20 minutes or until they are cooked through and browned on the outside.
5. For the glaze combine the olive oil, brown sugar, and balsamic vinegar in a small saucepan. Simmer over medium heat, cover, and cook until the mixture thickens and reduces by half, about 5-7 minutes.
6. Once the meatballs are done, drizzle the balsamic glaze over them or toss them in the glaze to coat evenly.
7. Serve the glazed meatballs warm, garnished with extra Parmesan or fresh herbs.

Roasted Chickpeas

Ingredients:

- 1 can (15 oz) of rinsed and drained chickpeas
- 1 tbsp olive oil
- 1/2 tsp paprika
- 1/4 tsp cumin
- 1/4 tsp dried oregano
- 1/4 tsp salt
- 1/8 tsp black pepper

Nutrition (per serving):

150 calories | 6g fat | 20g carbs | 6g protein | 2g sugar

Prep. time: 10 min **Total time:** 50 min **Servings:** 4

Directions:

1. Preheat your oven to 400°F (200°C).
2. Thoroughly dry the chickpeas with a towel.
3. Combine all the spices and olive oil with the chickpeas in a bowl until evenly coated.
4. On a baking sheet, arrange the chickpeas in a single layer.
5. Roast for 35 to 40 minutes in a preheated oven, shaking the pan every ten minutes until golden and crispy.
6. Take out of the oven and allow to cool a little before serving. Enjoy warm or keep for a few days in an airtight container.

Miso Soup with Tofu and Greens

Prep. time: 10 min | **Total time:** 20 min | **Servings:** 4

Ingredients:

- 4 cups water
- 2 tablespoons low FODMAP miso paste
- 1 cup firm tofu, diced
- 2 cups chopped spinach or other low FODMAP greens
- 1 tablespoon garlic-infused olive oil
- 1/2 teaspoon sesame oil
- 1/4 cup green onion tops, thinly sliced
- Optional: seaweed, sliced into small pieces

Directions:

1. In a medium pot, bring water to a simmer over medium heat.
2. In a small bowl, allow the miso paste to dissolve in a little hot water to make a smooth paste, then add it back to the pot.
3. Add the garlic-infused olive oil and sesame oil to the simmering water. Add the diced tofu and simmer for about 5 minutes.
4. Stir in the chopped greens and simmer for another 2-3 minutes until the greens are wilted but still vibrant.
5. Remove from heat and add the sliced green onion tops.
6. If using, add the seaweed just before serving.
7. Serve hot, ensuring each bowl is filled with equal amounts of tofu, greens, and flavorful broth.

Carrot Ginger Soup

Prep. time: 10 min | **Total time:** 40 min | **Servings:** 4

Ingredients:

- 1 pound carrots, peeled and chopped
- 1 tablespoon ginger, peeled and finely grated
- 2 tablespoons garlic-infused olive oil
- 4 cups low FODMAP vegetable broth
- Salt and pepper to taste
- 1/4 cup lactose-free cream
- Fresh parsley, chopped

Directions:

1. Heat the garlic-infused olive oil in a large pot over medium heat.
2. Add the chopped carrots and grated ginger to the pot, and sauté for about 5 minutes until the carrots start to soften.
3. After adding the veggie broth and bringing it to a boil, lower the heat to low and simmer for about 25 minutes, or until the carrots are very tender.
4. Purée the soup with a blender until smooth.
5. Add salt and pepper to taste. Serve hot, drizzled with lactose-free cream and chopped parsley.

Nutrition (per serving):

140 calories | 7g fat | 18g carbs | 2g protein | 9g sugar

Thai Coconut Chicken Soup

Ingredients:

- 1 tablespoon garlic-infused olive oil
- 1 pound chicken breast, thinly sliced
- 4 cups low FODMAP chicken broth
- 1 can (14 oz) coconut milk
- 1 tablespoon ginger, peeled and grated
- 1 tablespoon lime juice
- 2 teaspoons fish sauce
- 1/2 teaspoon sugar
- 1/2 teaspoon chili paste (ensure it's without garlic or onion)
- 1/2 cup chopped fresh cilantro
- 1/4 cup of chopped onion tops
- Salt to taste

Nutrition (per serving):

300 calories | 18g fat | 8g carbs | 28g protein | 3g sugar

Prep. time: 15 min   **Total time:** 35 min   **Servings:** 4

Directions:

1. In a large pot, warm the garlic-infused olive oil over medium heat.
2. Add the thinly sliced chicken breast and cook until it starts to turn white.
3. Pour in the low FODMAP chicken broth and coconut milk, bringing the mixture to a simmer.
4. Add the grated ginger, lime juice, fish sauce, sugar, and chili paste. Stir well to combine all the ingredients.
5. Reduce heat to low and simmer until the chicken is cooked through, about 15 minutes, and the flavors are well blended.
6. Stir in green onion tops and the chopped cilantro just before serving. Adjust seasoning with salt.
7. Serve hot, ensuring each bowl is fragrant with Thai flavors and enriched with creamy coconut milk.

Turkey and Rice Soup

Ingredients:

- 1 tablespoon garlic-infused olive oil
- 1 cup diced carrots
- 1/2 cup diced celery
- 1 cup cooked turkey, shredded or diced
- 1/2 cup cooked basmati rice
- 4 cups low FODMAP chicken or turkey broth
- 1 teaspoon dried thyme
- Salt and pepper to taste
- Fresh parsley, chopped (for garnish)

Nutrition (per serving):

200 calories | 5g fat | 20g carbs | 20g protein | 3g sugar

Prep. time: 15 min   **Total time:** 45 min   **Servings:** 4

Directions:

1. Heat the garlic-infused olive oil in a big saucepan over medium heat.
2. Add the diced carrots, celery, and sauté until vegetables soften (about 5 minutes).
3. Stir in the cooked turkey and cooked rice, mixing to combine.
4. Add the turkey or chicken broth and bring the mixture to a simmer.
5. Season the soup with dried thyme, salt, and pepper. Simmer for approximately 20-25 minutes to let the flavors blend.
6. Adjust seasoning as needed.
7. Serve hot, garnished with chopped fresh parsley.

Minestrone

Prep. time: 15 min   **Total time:** 45 min   **Servings:** 4

Ingredients:

- 1 tablespoon garlic-infused olive oil
- 1 cup diced carrots
- 1 cup diced zucchini
- 1/2 cup diced red bell pepper
- 1/2 cup green onion tops, sliced
- 1/2 cup of canned chickpeas, with liquid drained and rinsed
- 1/2 cup canned diced tomatoes (without onion or garlic)
- 4 cups low FODMAP vegetable broth
- 1 teaspoon dried basil
- 1 teaspoon dried oregano
- 1/2 cup gluten-free pasta (small)
- Salt and pepper to taste
- Fresh basil for garnish (optional)

Directions:

1. In a big pot, warm the garlic-infused olive oil over medium heat.
2. Add the diced carrots, zucchini and red bell pepper, sautéing for about 5 minutes until the vegetables start to soften.
3. Stir in the green onion tops, chickpeas, and diced tomatoes.
4. After adding the vegetable broth, boil the mixture.
5. Salt and pepper to taste. Add the dried oregano and basil.
6. Stir in the gluten-free pasta and continue to simmer for 10-15 minutes or until the pasta is tender.
7. Adjust the seasoning and top hot dish with freshly chopped basil if desired.

Nutrition (per serving):

180 calories | 4g fat | 32g carbs | 6g protein | 4g sugar

Pumpkin Soup

Prep. time: 15 min   **Total time:** 45 min   **Servings:** 4

Ingredients:

- 2 tablespoons garlic-infused olive oil
- 1 medium pumpkin, peeled, seeded, and chopped (about 4 cups)
- 4 cups low FODMAP vegetable broth
- 1 teaspoon ground ginger
- 1/2 teaspoon ground nutmeg
- Salt and pepper to taste
- 1/4 cup lactose-free cream for garnish (optional)
- Fresh chives, chopped (for garnish)

Directions:

1. Warm the garlic-infused olive oil in a large pot over medium heat.
2. Add the chopped pumpkin to the pot and sauté for about 10 minutes until it begins to soften.
3. Add the vegetable broth and heat until it boils. Reduce heat to low and simmer for about 20 minutes or until the pumpkin becomes tender all the way through.
4. Add the ground ginger and nutmeg, then season with salt and pepper to taste.
5. Smooth the soup directly in the pot by using a blender.
6. Serve hot, drizzled with lactose-free cream and garnished with chopped chives if desired.

Moroccan Spiced Vegetable Soup

Ingredients:

- 1 tablespoon garlic-infused olive oil
- 1 cup diced carrots
- 1 cup diced zucchini
- 1/2 cup diced red bell pepper
- 4 cups low FODMAP vegetable broth
- 1 teaspoon ground cumin
- 1 teaspoon ground coriander
- 1/2 teaspoon ground cinnamon
- 1/2 teaspoon ground turmeric
- 1 can (14.5 oz) diced tomatoes (ensure no onion or garlic is added)
- Salt and pepper to taste
- 1/4 cup of fresh chopped cilantro (for garnishing)
- 1/4 cup cooked quinoa (optional, for serving)

Prep. time: 10 min **Total time:** 30 min **Servings:** 4

Directions:

1. Heat the garlic-infused olive oil in a big pot over medium heat.
2. Add the diced carrots, zucchini, and red bell pepper, and sauté for about 5 minutes until the vegetables begin to soften.
3. Stir in the ground cinnamon, coriander, cumin and turmeric, cooking for another minute until the spices are fragrant.
4. Add the diced tomatoes and veggie broth, and bring the soup to a boil.
5. After lowering the heat, simmer the soup for around 20 minutes, or until the vegetables are tender.
6. Season with salt and pepper to taste.
7. If using, add cooked quinoa to each bowl for added texture.
8. Serve the soup hot, garnished with chopped fresh cilantro.

Nutrition (per serving):

150 calories | 5g fat | 23g carbs | 5g protein | 7g sugar

Zucchini Cream Soup

Ingredients:

- 1 tablespoon garlic-infused olive oil
- 4 medium zucchinis, chopped
- 4 cups low FODMAP vegetable broth
- Salt and pepper to taste
- 1/4 cup lactose-free cream (optional, for serving)
- Fresh basil or parsley, chopped (for garnish)

Prep. time: 10 min **Total time:** 30 min **Servings:** 4

Directions:

1. Heat the garlic-infused olive oil in a big pot over medium heat.
2. Add the chopped zucchini and sauté for about 5 minutes, stirring occasionally, until slightly softened.
3. After adding the veggie broth, heat the mixture until it boils. Simmer for around 15 minutes on low heat or until the zucchini is very tender.
4. Purée until in a blender until smooth.
5. Add salt and pepper to taste.
6. If using, stir in the lactose-free cream for a richer texture and reheat gently without boiling.
7. Garnish with chopped fresh basil or parsley and serve hot.

Nutrition (per serving):

90 calories | 5g fat | 10g carbs | 3g protein | 5g sugar

Vegetable Broth

Ingredients:

- 2 tablespoons garlic-infused olive oil
- 2 carrots, peeled and roughly chopped
- 2 parsnips, peeled and roughly chopped
- 1 FODMAP-friendly leek (green part only), roughly chopped
- 1/2 a fennel bulb, roughly chopped
- 1 red bell pepper, roughly cut and deseeded
- 1/2 cup chopped green onion tops
- 1/2 cup fresh parsley
- 10 cups water
- 2 bay leaves
- 1 teaspoon peppercorns
- Salt to taste

Prep. time: 10 min   **Total time:** 1 hr 10 min   **Servings:** 4

Directions:

1. In a large pot, heat the garlic-infused olive oil over medium heat.
2. Add the carrots, parsnips, leek greens, fennel, and red bell pepper to the pot and sauté them for about five minutes, or until they start to get tender and release their flavors.
3. Add the green onion tops and parsley, stirring to combine.
4. After adding the water, add the bay leaves and peppercorns.
5. Lower the heat after the mixture reaches a boiling point and simmer, uncovered, for approximately one hour.
6. Pour the broth through a sieve with fine mesh, applying pressure to the veggies to extract as much liquid as possible. Discard the solids.
7. Season the broth with salt to taste.
8. Use the broth immediately, or let it fully cool before placing it in the fridge or freezer for later use.

Lentil Soup with Carrots and Kale

Ingredients:

- 1 tablespoon garlic-infused olive oil
- 1 cup carrots, diced
- 1 cup canned lentils, rinsed and drained
- 4 cups low FODMAP vegetable broth
- 2 cups chopped kale, stems removed
- 1 teaspoon dried thyme
- Salt and pepper to taste
- Fresh parsley, chopped (for garnish)

Prep. time: 15 min   **Total time:** 60 min   **Servings:** 4

Nutrition (per serving):

180 calories | 4g fat | 25g carbs | 12g protein | 5g sugar

Directions:

1. Heat the garlic-infused olive oil in a large pot over medium heat.
2. Add the diced carrots and sauté until they begin to soften, about 5 minutes.
3. Stir the washed lentils into the carrot mixture.
4. After adding the vegetable broth, raise the temperature to a boil. Next, turn down the heat and simmer it for half an hour.
5. Stir in the chopped kale and dried thyme, and continue to simmer for another 15 minutes, or until the kale is tender.
6. Season with salt and pepper to taste.
7. Serve hot, garnished with chopped fresh parsley.

Seafood Chowder

Prep. time: 15 min　　**Total time:** 40 min　　**Servings:** 4

Ingredients:

- 1 tablespoon garlic-infused olive oil
- 1 cup diced carrots
- 1 cup diced potatoes
- 1/2 cup chopped green onion tops
- 4 cups low FODMAP fish or seafood broth
- 1 cup lactose-free cream
- 1 pound mixed seafood (such as shrimp, scallops, and firm white fish), chopped into bite-sized pieces
- 1 teaspoon dried thyme
- Salt and pepper to taste
- Fresh parsley, chopped (for garnish)

Directions:

1. Warm the garlic-infused olive oil in a big saucepan over medium heat.
2. Add the diced carrots and potatoes, sautéing for about 5 minutes until they start to soften.
3. Stir in the chopped green onion tops and sauté for another 2 minutes.
4. Add the seafood or fish broth and heat the mixture until it boils. Reduce heat to a simmer and cook for about 10 minutes or until the vegetables are tender.
5. Stir in the mixed seafood and dried thyme. Simmer for another 5 minutes or until the seafood is cooked through.
6. Reduce heat to low and stir in the lactose-free cream. Heat gently, avoiding boiling, until the chowder is hot and creamy. Season with salt and pepper to taste.
7. Garnish the hot chowder with finely chopped fresh parsley.

Nutrition (per serving):

310 calories | 12g fat | 25g carbs | 25g protein | 4g sugar

Chapter 4: Salads and Sides
Carrot and Walnut Salad

Prep. time: 10 min **Total time:** 10 min **Servings:** 4

Ingredients:
- 4 large carrots, peeled and grated
- 1 cup walnuts, chopped
- 1/4 cup raisins
- 2 tablespoons olive oil
- 2 tablespoons lemon juice
- 1 teaspoon honey
- Salt and pepper to taste
- Fresh parsley, chopped (optional for garnish)

Directions:
1. Combine chopped walnuts, grated carrots and raisins in a big bowl.
2. Whisk together lemon juice, olive oil, salt, honey and pepper to create the dressing in a small bowl.
3. Add the dressing over the carrot mixture and toss to coat everything evenly.
4. Before serving, let the salad stay in the fridge for at least 30 minutes to let the flavors to merge.
5. Use fresh parsley to garnish before serving if desired.

Nutrition (per serving):
280 calories | 20g fat | 24g carbs | 4g protein | 12g sugar

Egg Salad with Dill

Prep. time: 10 min **Total time:** 20 min **Servings:** 4

Ingredients:
- 8 large eggs, hard-boiled and peeled
- 1/4 cup mayonnaise
- 1 tablespoon Dijon mustard
- 1/4 cup fresh dill, finely chopped
- Salt and pepper to taste

Directions:
1. Finely chop the hard-boiled eggs into pieces and place them in a large mixing bowl.
2. Add the mayonnaise, Dijon mustard, and chopped dill to the eggs. Season with salt and pepper.
3. Combine all the ingredients, mixing gently until creamy.
4. Serve it once or refrigerate to let the flavors merge together. Egg salad can be served as a filling for sandwiches, over a bed of lettuce or on its own.

Nutrition (per serving):
230 calories | 18g fat | 1g carbs | 13g protein | 0g sugar

Quinoa Tabbouleh

Ingredients:

- 1 cup quinoa, uncooked
- 2 cups water
- 1 cup fresh, finely chopped parsley
- 1/2 cup fresh, finely chopped mint leaves
- 1 cucumber, diced
- 1 cup cherry tomatoes, halved
- 1/4 cup lemon juice
- 1/4 cup olive oil
- Salt and pepper to taste

Nutrition (per serving):

290 calories | 15g fat | 35g carbs | 6g protein | 4g sugar

Prep. time: 15 min   **Total time:** 30 min   **Servings:** 4

Directions:

1. Rinse the quinoa in cool water until the water becomes clear.
2. Bring the two cups of water to a boil in a medium-sized pot. After adding quinoa, lower the heat to a simmer, cover, and let the quinoa cook for 15 minutes, or until it is tender and the water is absorbed.
3. After turning off the heat, leave the quinoa covered for five minutes. Using a fork, fluff the mixture and let it cool to room temperature.
4. Combine the quinoa, chopped mint, parsley, cucumber, and cherry tomatoes in a large bowl.
5. Mix salt, lemon juice, olive oil and pepper in a small bowl. Add the dressing over the quinoa mixture and toss to combine thoroughly.
6. Chill in the refrigerator to let the flavors merge for 60 minutes before serving. Serve chilled.

Arugula and Shaved Parmesan Salad

Ingredients:

- 6 cups arugula, washed and dried
- 1/2 cup shaved Parmesan cheese
- 1/4 cup pine nuts, toasted
- 2 tablespoons extra virgin olive oil
- 1 tablespoon lemon juice
- Salt and pepper to taste

Nutrition (per serving):

200 calories | 17g fat | 3g carbs | 8g protein | 1g sugar

Prep. time: 10 min   **Total time:** 10 min   **Servings:** 4

Directions:

1. Combine the arugula, shaved Parmesan, and toasted pine nuts in a large salad bowl.
2. Whisk together lemon juice and the olive oil in a small bowl. Season with salt and pepper to taste.
3. Toss the salad gently after adding the dressing to combine all the ingredients.
4. Serve right away, with a taste that is both spicy and fresh, enhanced by the savory and nutty undertones of pine nuts and Parmesan cheese.

Roasted Potato Salad

Ingredients:

- 2 pounds small red potatoes
- 3 tablespoons garlic-infused olive oil
- Salt and pepper to taste
- 1/4 cup fresh dill, chopped
- 1/4 cup green onions (green parts only), chopped
- 2 tablespoons Dijon mustard
- 2 tablespoons apple cider vinegar

Nutrition (per serving):

280 calories | 11g fat | 40g carbs | 5g protein | 4g sugar

Prep. time: 10 min **Total time:** 35 min **Servings:** 4

Directions:

1. Preheat your oven to 425°F (220°C).
2. Toss the quartered red potatoes with 2 tablespoons of garlic-infused olive oil, salt and pepper.
3. Arrange the potatoes on a baking sheet in one layer.
4. Roast, tossing halfway through, in a preheated oven for about 25 minutes or until golden and crispy.
5. In a large bowl, whisk together the remaining 1 tablespoon of olive oil, Dijon mustard, apple cider vinegar, chopped dill, and green onions. Add the roasted potatoes while still warm to the dressing and toss to coat evenly.
6. Add additional salt and pepper if needed.
7. Serve warm or at room temperature.

Zucchini Noodle Salad

Ingredients:

- 4 medium zucchinis, spiralized
- 1 carrot, spiralized
- 1 red bell pepper, thinly sliced
- 1/4 cup chopped peanuts
- 1/4 cup fresh cilantro, chopped
- 1/4 cup fresh lime juice
- 2 tablespoons sesame oil
- 1 tablespoon soy sauce
- 1 tablespoon honey
- 1 teaspoon red pepper flakes (optional, to taste)

Prep. time: 15 min **Total time:** 15 min **Servings:** 4

Directions:

1. Combine the spiralized zucchini, carrot, and thinly sliced red bell pepper in a large bowl.
2. In a small bowl, thoroughly whisk together the soy sauce, honey, sesame oil, lime juice and red pepper flakes.
3. Drizzle the dressing over the mixture of zucchini noodles and toss to coat evenly.
4. Sprinkle with chopped peanuts and fresh cilantro.
5. Serve immediately, or let it stay in the refrigerator for about 10 minutes to let the flavors meld together.

Nutrition (per serving):

180 calories | 10g fat | 20g carbs | 4g protein | 10g sugar

Rice Salad with Fennel and Orange

Ingredients:

- 1 cup basmati rice
- 2 cups water
- 1 fennel bulb, thinly sliced
- 2 oranges, peeled and segments cut into pieces
- 1/4 cup sliced almonds, toasted
- 1/4 cup fresh parsley, chopped
- 3 tablespoons olive oil
- 1 tablespoon white wine vinegar
- Salt and pepper to taste

Nutrition (per serving):

300 calories | 11g fat | 44g carbs | 6g protein | 5g sugar

Prep. time: 15 min   **Total time:** 30   **Servings:** 4

Directions:

1. Rinse the basmati rice under cold water until it runs clear.
2. Place two cups of water in a medium pot and boil. Add the rice, lower the heat, cover, and simmer for 15 minutes or until the water is absorbed and the rice is tender.
3. Remove the pan from the heat and let it sit, covered, for 5 minutes. Fluff the rice with a fork and let it cool to room temperature.
4. In a large bowl, combine the rice with thinly sliced fennel, orange segments, toasted almonds, and chopped parsley.
5. Mix the olive oil, white wine vinegar, salt, and pepper.
6. Pour the dressing over the rice mixture and toss to mix thoroughly.
7. Keep in the refrigerator for at least 1 hour before serving to let the flavors blend. Serve chilled.

Mini Caprese Salad

Ingredients:

- 1 pint cherry tomatoes, halved
- 8 oz fresh lactose-free mozzarella cheese, sliced into little cubes
- 1/4 cup fresh basil leaves, chopped
- 2 tablespoons garlic-infused olive oil
- 1 tablespoon balsamic vinegar
- Salt and pepper to taste

Prep. time: 10 min   **Total time:** 10 min   **Servings:** 4

Directions:

1. In a medium bowl, combine cherry tomatoes, cubed mozzarella, and chopped basil.
2. Drizzle with garlic-infused olive oil and balsamic vinegar.
3. Gently toss to combine all the ingredients. Season with salt and pepper to taste.
4. Serve right away.

Nutrition (per serving):

220 calories | 16g fat | 6g carbs | 14g protein | 4g sugar

Grilled Chicken Caesar Salad

Ingredients:

- 2 boneless, skinless chicken breasts
- 1 teaspoon olive oil
- Salt and pepper to taste
- 8 cups chopped romaine lettuce
- 1/2 cup grated Parmesan cheese
- 1 cup croutons (gluten-free)
- Caesar dressing (low FODMAP)

Nutrition (per serving):

310 calories | 16g fat | 12g carbs | 28g protein | 2g sugar

Prep. time: 15 min **Total time:** 25 min **Servings:** 4

Directions:

1. Preheat the grill to medium-high heat.
2. Add some pepper and salt to the chicken breasts after brushing them with olive oil. Grill the chicken for about 5 minutes per side, or until it is fully cooked and the internal temperature reaches 165°F (74°C).
3. Let the chicken rest for a few minutes, then slice it thinly.
4. In a large bowl, mix the chopped romaine lettuce with Caesar dressing, coating the leaves evenly.
5. Toss the salad gently after adding the croutons and grated Parmesan cheese.
6. Divide the salad among four plates and top each with sliced grilled chicken.
7. Serve immediately.

Garlic-Infused Olive Oil Sautéed Spinach

Ingredients:

- 8 cups fresh spinach
- 2 tablespoons garlic-infused olive oil
- Salt and pepper to taste
- Lemon wedges for serving (optional)

Nutrition (per serving):

60 calories | 5g fat | 3g carbs | 2g protein | 1g sugar

Prep. time: 5 min **Total time:** 10 min **Servings:** 4

Directions:

1. Place a big skillet over medium heat and add the garlic-infused olive oil.
2. In batches, add the spinach to the frying pan, tossing frequently until the spinach wilts, about 1-2 minutes per batch.
3. Once all the spinach has been wilted and added to the skillet, season with salt and pepper, and sauté all together for an additional minute to blend the flavors.
4. Serve right away with lemon slices on the side for a fresh, tangy squeeze.

Pumpkin and Spinach Salad

Ingredients:

- 2 cups pumpkin, peeled and diced
- 3 tablespoons garlic-infused olive oil
- Salt and pepper to taste
- 4 cups baby spinach leaves
- 1/2 cup toasted pine nuts
- 1/4 cup crumbled feta cheese (lactose-free if necessary)
- 2 tablespoons balsamic vinegar

Nutrition (per serving):

280 calories | 23g fat | 14g carbs | 5g protein | 5g sugar

Prep. time: 15 min   **Total time:** 35   **Servings:** 4

Directions:

1. Preheat your oven to 400°F (200°C).
2. Toss the diced pumpkin with 1 tablespoon olive oil, salt, and pepper. Spread out on a baking sheet in a single layer.
3. Roast in the preheated oven for about 20 minutes, or until tender and lightly caramelized, stirring halfway through.
4. Allow the roasted pumpkin to cool slightly.
5. Combine the cooled pumpkin, baby spinach, toasted pine nuts, and crumbled feta cheese in a large salad bowl.
6. Whisk the extra virgin olive oil and the balsamic vinegar in a small bowl. Pore over the salad and gently toss to mix.
7. Serve the salad immediately or chill briefly in the refrigerator before serving to blend the flavors.

Cucumber and Radish Salad

Ingredients:

- 2 large cucumbers, thinly sliced
- 1 cup radishes, thinly sliced
- 1/4 cup rice vinegar
- 2 tablespoons olive oil
- 1 tablespoon maple syrup
- Salt and pepper to taste
- 2 tablespoons fresh dill, chopped

Nutrition (per serving):

100 calories | 7g fat | 10g carbs | 1g protein | 5g sugar

Prep. time: 10 min   **Total time:** 10 min   **Servings:** 4

Directions:

1. Combine the thinly sliced cucumbers and radishes in a big bowl.
2. Whisk together the maple syrup, rice vinegar, olive oil, salt and pepper for the dressing.
3. Add the dressing over the radish and cucumber slices, tossing gently to coat evenly.
4. Keep the salad in the refrigerator for at least 30 minutes to let the flavors merge.
5. Right before serving, sprinkle with chopped fresh dill for an added burst of flavor.

Broccoli and Bacon Salad

Ingredients:

- 4 cups broccoli florets
- 6 slices bacon, cooked and crumbled
- 1/4 cup sunflower seeds
- 1/4 cup raisins (optional)
- 1/2 cup mayonnaise (lactose-free)
- 2 tablespoons apple cider vinegar
- 1 tablespoon sugar
- Salt and pepper to taste

Nutrition (per serving):

320 calories | 28g fat | 12g carbs | 7g protein | 6g sugar

Prep. time: 15 min   **Total time:** 25 min   **Servings:** 4

Directions:

1. Boil some water and blanch the broccoli florets for about 2 minutes, just until they are bright green and slightly tender. Drain and rinse under cold water.
2. Add the blanched broccoli to a large mixing bowl, crumbled bacon, sunflower seeds, and raisins if using.
3. In a small bowl, whisk together the mayonnaise, apple cider vinegar, sugar, salt and pepper.
4. Cover the broccoli mixture with the dressing and toss to coat evenly.
5. Before serving, chill in the refrigerator for at least 60 minutes to let the flavors meld.

Stir-Fried Bell Peppers

Ingredients:

- 3 bell peppers thinly sliced
- 1 tablespoon garlic-infused olive oil
- 2 tablespoons soy sauce
- 1 tablespoon ginger, grated
- 1 tablespoon sesame oil
- 1/4 teaspoon chili flakes (optional)
- 2 tablespoons green onion tops, sliced
- 1 tablespoon sesame seeds

Nutrition (per serving):

110 calories | 7g fat | 10g carbs | 2g protein | 6g sugar

Prep. time: 10 min   **Total time:** 20 min   **Servings:** 4

Directions:

1. Warm the garlic-infused olive oil in a big skillet or wok over medium-high heat.
2. Thinly slice bell peppers, add to the pan, and stir-fry for about 5-7 minutes or until they are tender-crisp.
3. Stir in the soy sauce, finely grated ginger, sesame oil, and chili flakes if using. Simmer for a further two to three minutes to let the flavors combine.
4. Remove from heat and sprinkle the sliced green onion tops over the cooked bell peppers.
5. Add sesame seeds for garnishing if desired and serve immediately.

Spinach and Cheese Stuffed Potatoes

Ingredients:

- 4 large russet potatoes
- 2 tablespoons garlic-infused olive oil
- 2 cups fresh spinach, chopped
- 1/2 cup lactose-free sour cream
- 1/2 cup grated cheddar cheese (lactose-free if necessary)
- Salt and pepper to taste
- 2 tablespoons chives, chopped (green parts only)

Nutrition (per serving):

320 calories | 12g fat | 42g carbs | 8g protein | 3g sugar

Prep. time: 10 min **Total time:** 1 hr 20 min **Servings:** 4

Directions:

1. Preheat your oven to 400°F (200°C).
2. After washing, give the potatoes several fork pricks. Place them directly on the oven rack and bake for 1 hour or until soft.
3. While the potatoes are baking, heat the garlic-infused olive oil in a skillet over medium heat. Add the spinach and sauté until wilted, about 2-3 minutes. Set aside to cool slightly.
4. Once the potatoes are done, let them cool slightly before slicing the top off of each potato. Carefully scoop out most of the flesh, preserving the structure by keeping a thin layer affixed to the skin.
5. Mash the removed potato flesh with the sour cream in a bowl. Stir in the sautéed spinach, cheddar cheese, and season with salt and pepper.
6. Return the mixture to the potato skins with a spoon.
7. Return the stuffed potatoes to the oven and continue baking for ten more minutes or until the cheese has melted and the tops are brown.
8. Garnish with chopped chives and serve hot.

Sautéed Broccoli with Garlic Oil

Ingredients:

- 4 cups broccoli florets
- 2 tablespoons garlic-infused olive oil
- Salt and pepper to taste
- 1 tablespoon lemon juice (optional)
- 1/4 cup grated Parmesan cheese (lactose-free if necessary)

Nutrition (per serving):

120 calories | 9g fat | 7g carbs | 5g protein | 2g sugar

Prep. time: 5 min **Total time:** 15 min **Servings:** 4

Directions:

1. In a large skillet, heat the garlic-infused olive oil over medium heat.
2. After adding the broccoli florets to the skillet, cook them for 5 to 7 minutes or until the broccoli is bright green and tender. Stir frequently to ensure even cooking.
3. Season with salt and pepper to taste, and if using, drizzle with lemon juice for a zesty flavor.
4. Sprinkle grated Parmesan cheese over the broccoli just before serving.
5. Serve hot as a tasty and nourishing side dish.

Butternut Squash Risotto

Ingredients:

- 2 cups butternut squash, peeled and cubed
- 1 tablespoon olive oil
- 4 cups low FODMAP chicken or vegetable broth
- 1 cup arborio rice
- 1/2 cup dry white wine
- 2 tablespoons garlic-infused olive oil
- 1/2 cup grated Parmesan cheese
- Salt and pepper to taste
- Fresh sage leaves, finely chopped (optional, for garnish)

Nutrition (per serving):

380 calories | 12g fat | 54g carbs | 10g protein | 3g sugar

Prep. time: 15 min **Total time:** 55 min **Servings:** 4

Directions:

1. Preheat your oven to 400°F (200°C). Add a little salt, pepper and olive oil to the butternut squash cubes and toss them. Place on a baking sheet and roast for 20-25 minutes or until soft and lightly caramelized.
2. Keep the chicken or vegetable broth warm over low heat in a saucepan.
3. In another large saucepan, heat the garlic-infused olive oil over medium heat. When the arborio rice is added, stir to coat the grains in oil. Cook for 1-2 minutes more until the edges of the grains become slightly translucent.
4. Add the white wine and stir constantly until the rice has absorbed most of the wine.
5. One ladle at a time, add the heated broth, stirring constantly and letting each addition absorb before adding the next. Continue this process until the rice is creamy and just tender, about 25-30 minutes.
6. Stir in the roasted butternut squash and grated Parmesan cheese. Season with salt and pepper to taste.
7. Serve immediately, garnished with fresh sage if desired.

Chicken and Orange Salad

Ingredients:

- 2 boneless, skinless chicken breasts
- 1 tablespoon olive oil
- Salt and pepper to taste
- 3 oranges, peeled and segmented
- 1/4 cup chopped walnuts, toasted
- 4 cups mixed arugula and spinach
- 1/4 cup chopped fresh chives

Dressing:
- 3 tablespoons extra virgin olive oil
- 1 tablespoon white wine vinegar
- 1 tablespoon Dijon mustard (make sure it's low FODMAP)
- 1 teaspoon orange zest
- Salt and pepper to taste

Prep. time: 15 min **Total time:** 30 min **Servings:** 4

Directions:

1. Toss the chicken breasts with a bit of salt and pepper. Warm up one tablespoon of olive oil in a skillet over medium heat. Cook the chicken for about 7 minutes per side until golden and cooked through. Let it cool, then slice thinly.
2. Mix the salad greens, orange segments, sliced chicken, toasted walnuts, and chives in a large salad bowl.
3. Whisk together Dijon mustard, white wine vinegar, olive oil, orange zest, salt, and pepper to create the dressing in a small bowl.
4. Add the dressing over the salad, then mix gently to combine all the ingredients.
5. Serve immediately, ensuring that the flavors remain fresh and vibrant.

Nutrition (per serving):

310 calories | 19g fat | 16g carbs | 22g protein | 10g sugar

Roasted Red Cabbage Steaks

Ingredients:

- 1 medium red cabbage
- 2 tablespoons garlic-infused olive oil
- 2 tablespoons balsamic vinegar
- Salt and pepper to taste
- 1 teaspoon dried thyme

Nutrition (per serving):

110 calories | 7g fat | 12g carbs | 2g protein | 7g sugar

Prep. time: 10 min **Total time:** 35 min **Servings:** 4

Directions:

1. Preheat your oven to 400°F (200°C). Line a baking sheet with parchment paper.
2. Slice the red cabbage into 1-inch thick slices, ensuring each slice remains intact as a "steak.".
3. Brush each side of cabbage steaks with garlic-infused olive oil and balsamic vinegar. Season with salt, pepper, and dried thyme.
4. Arrange the cabbage steaks on the prepared baking sheet in a single layer.
5. Roast in the preheated oven for nearly 12-15 minutes on each side, until the cabbage is tender and the edges start to crisp up.
6. Serve hot, with additional balsamic vinegar drizzled over the top.

Ratatouille

Ingredients:

- 1 medium zucchini, sliced into rounds
- 1 medium yellow squash, sliced into rounds
- 1 medium eggplant, sliced into rounds
- 1 red bell pepper, thinly sliced and deseeded
- 1 can (14 oz) diced tomatoes (no added onion or garlic)
- 2 tablespoons garlic-infused olive oil
- 1 teaspoon dried thyme
- 1 teaspoon dried basil
- Salt and pepper to taste
- 1/4 cup fresh, chopped basil (for garnish)

Prep. time: 20 min **Total time:** 60 min **Servings:** 4

Directions:

1. Preheat your oven to 375°F (190°C).
2. Spread the diced tomatoes in the bottom of a large baking dish. Stir in the garlic-infused olive oil, dried thyme, and dried basil. Season with salt and pepper.
3. Arrange the sliced vegetables (zucchini, yellow squash, eggplant, and red bell pepper) in a spiral pattern or neat rows over the tomato base, alternating and packing them tightly.
4. Bake the dish covered with foil in a preheated oven for 30 minutes. Remove the foil after 30 minutes and continue baking for 10 minutes more or until the vegetables are tender.
5. Garnish with fresh chopped basil before serving.

Nutrition (per serving):

150 calories | 7g fat | 21g carbs | 4g protein | 12g sugar

Grilled Zucchini Ribbons

Ingredients:

- 4 large zucchinis
- 2 tablespoons garlic-infused olive oil
- Salt and pepper to taste
- 1/4 cup freshly grated Parmesan cheese
- 1 tablespoon chopped fresh basil

Prep. time: 10 min **Total time:** 15 min **Servings:** 4

Nutrition (per serving):

120 calories | 9g fat | 7g carbs | 4g protein | 3g sugar

Directions:

1. Preheat your grill to medium-high heat.
2. Slice the zucchinis lengthwise into thin ribbons with a mandoline or vegetable peeler.
3. Toss the zucchini ribbons with garlic-infused olive oil, salt, and pepper.
4. Grill the zucchini ribbons for about 2-3 minutes on each side or until they are tender and have grill marks.
5. Place the grilled zucchini on a serving plate. Add chopped basil and freshly grated Parmesan cheese on top.
6. Serve immediately.

Lactose-Free Potato Gratin

Ingredients:

- 2 pounds Yukon Gold potatoes, thinly sliced
- 1 cup lactose-free heavy cream
- 2 cups grated cheddar cheese (lactose-free)
- 2 tablespoons garlic-infused olive oil
- 1 teaspoon dried thyme
- Salt and pepper to taste

Nutrition (per serving):

350 calories | 22g fat | 30g carbs | 10g protein | 3g sugar

Prep. time: 20 min **Total time:** 1hr 20 min **Servings:** 6

Directions:

1. Preheat the oven to 375°F (190°C). Apply garlic-infused olive oil to a 9 x 13-inch baking dish.
2. Lay potato slices at the bottom of the dish. Drizzle with a bit more garlic-infused olive oil, sprinkle with some thyme, salt, and pepper.
3. Pour a small amount of lactose-free heavy cream over the potatoes and sprinkle a layer of grated cheddar cheese.
4. Make the next layer with potatoes, cream, finishing with a cheese layer on top for a golden crust.
5. Bake the dish covered with aluminum foil in the preheated oven for 1 hour.
6. After removing the foil bake for an additional 15-20 minutes, or until the top is bubbly and golden brown.
7. Before serving, let the gratin settle for ten minutes.

Green Beans with Toasted Almonds

Ingredients:

- 1 pound green beans, trimmed
- 1/4 cup sliced almonds
- 2 tablespoons olive oil
- Salt and pepper to taste
- Lemon zest from 1 lemon (optional for extra flavor)

Nutrition (per serving):

150 calories | 11g fat | 10g carbs | 4g protein | 3g sugar

Prep. time: 10 min **Total time:** 20 min **Servings:** 4

Directions:

1. Boil water in a large pot. Add the green beans and simmer for about 5 minutes until they are bright green and tender-crisp. Drain and place them into ice water. Drain again and set aside.
2. Toast the sliced almonds over medium heat in a dry skillet until aromatic and golden brown. Remove from heat and set aside.
3. Heat the olive oil in the same skillet. Add the drained green beans and sauté for 2-3 minutes, or until they are heated through.
4. If using, add the zest of one lemon and season with salt and pepper.
5. Place the green beans on a platter for serving and sprinkle with the toasted almonds. Serve immediately.

Quinoa and Vegetable Stuffed Peppers

Prep. time: 20 min   **Total time:** 50 min   **Servings:** 4

Ingredients:

- 4 large bell peppers, tops cut off and seeds removed
- 1 cup quinoa, cooked
- 1 tablespoon garlic-infused olive oil
- 1 zucchini, diced
- 1 carrot, diced
- 1 cup spinach, chopped
- 1/2 cup canned corn, drained (ensure it's low FODMAP if canned with other ingredients)
- 1 cup grated lactose-free cheddar cheese
- Salt and pepper to taste

Nutrition (per serving):

320 calories | 15g fat | 36g carbs | 12g protein | 5g sugar

Directions:

1. Preheat your oven to 375°F (190°C).
2. Heat the garlic-infused olive oil in a skillet over medium heat. Add the diced zucchini and carrot, sautéing until tender, about 5-7 minutes.
3. Stir in the chopped spinach and corn, simmering for two to three minutes or until the spinach has wilted.
4. Take away from heat and add the cooked quinoa. Season with salt and pepper.
5. Stir in half of the grated cheese into the quinoa and vegetable mixture until well combined.
6. Stuff the prepared bell peppers with the quinoa mixture, packing them firmly.
7. Lay the stuffed peppers in a baking dish. Sprinkle the tops with the remaining cheese.
8. Bake for around 30 minutes in the preheated oven, or until the peppers are soft and the cheese is melted and slightly golden.
9. Serve hot, ideally with a side salad or crusty bread for a complete meal

Chapter 5: Poultry, Meat and Seafood
Grilled Chicken with Herbs

Ingredients:

- 4 boneless, skinless chicken breasts
- 2 tablespoons garlic-infused olive oil
- 1 tablespoon fresh rosemary
- 1 tablespoon fresh thyme
- 1 tablespoon fresh parsley
- Salt and pepper to taste
- Lemon wedges, for serving

Nutrition (per serving):

220 calories | 7g fat | 1g carbs | 35g protein | 0g sugar

Prep. time: 15 min **Total time:** 30 min **Servings:** 4

Directions:

1. Preheat your grill to medium-high heat.
2. Apply garlic-infused olive oil to the chicken breasts.
3. In a small bowl, mix together the chopped rosemary, thyme, parsley, salt, and pepper.
4. Rub the herb mixture all over the chicken breasts, ensuring they are well-coated.
5. Place the chicken on the grill and cook for about 7-8 minutes on each side, or until the chicken is fully cooked and has nice grill marks (the internal temperature should reach 165°F or 74°C).
6. Take the chicken off the grill and set it aside to rest for a few minutes before slicing.
7. Serve the chicken hot, with freshly cut lemon wedges for squeezing over it.

Rosemary Infused Roast Beef

Ingredients:

- 2 pounds beef roast (such as sirloin tip or rump roast)
- 2 tablespoons garlic-infused olive oil
- 2 tablespoons fresh rosemary, finely chopped
- Salt and pepper to taste
- 1/2 cup low FODMAP beef broth

Nutrition (per serving):

450 calories | 25g fat | 0g carbs | 55g protein | 0g sugar

Prep. time: 10 min **Total time:** 1 hr 10 min **Servings:** 4

Directions:

1. Preheat your oven to 375°F (190°C).
2. Rub the beef roast all over with garlic-infused olive oil.
3. Season generously with chopped rosemary, salt, and pepper, pressing the herbs and seasonings into the surface of the meat to adhere.
4. Add the roast and the beef broth to the pan.
5. Roast in the preheated oven for about 1 hour until medium rare or until a meat thermometer in the thickest part of the roast registers 135°F (57°C)
6. Remove the roast from the oven and let it sit for at least 10 minutes before slicing. This helps the juices to spread evenly throughout the meat, making it juicy and flavorful.
7. Cut the roast thinly against the grain for serving.

Maple Mustard Pork Chops

Ingredients:

- 4 pork chops, 1-inch thick
- Salt and pepper to taste
- 2 tablespoons garlic-infused olive oil
- 1/4 cup Dijon mustard (ensure it's low FODMAP)
- 3 tablespoons pure maple syrup
- 1 tablespoon apple cider vinegar
- 1 teaspoon dried thyme

Nutrition (per serving):

320 calories | 15g fat | 15g carbs | 30g protein | 10g sugar

Prep. time: 10 min **Total time:** 25 min **Servings:** 4

Directions:

1. Add salt and pepper to each side of the pork chops.
2. In a large skillet, heat the garlic-infused olive oil over medium-high heat.
3. Place the pork chops in the skillet and cook for about 5-7 minutes on each side until golden brown and cooked through (internal temperature should reach 145°F).
4. Whisk the Dijon mustard, apple cider vinegar, maple syrup, and dried thyme in a small bowl.
5. Once the pork chops are cooked, reduce the heat to low and cover them in the skillet with the maple mustard mixture.
6. Continue cooking for 2-3 more minutes, spooning the sauce over the pork chops to glaze them thoroughly.
7. Serve the pork chops hot, drizzled with the remaining sauce from the skillet.

Lemon Herb Roast Chicken

Ingredients:

- 1 whole chicken (about 4 pounds)
- 2 tablespoons garlic-infused olive oil
- 1 lemon, cut into quarters
- 2 tablespoons chopped fresh rosemary
- 2 tablespoons chopped fresh thyme
- 1 tablespoon chopped fresh parsley
- 1 teaspoon salt
- 1/2 teaspoon black pepper
- 1 cup low FODMAP chicken broth

Prep. time: 20 min **Total time:** 1 hr 50 min **Servings:** 6

Directions:

1. Preheat the oven to 375°F (190°C).
2. Rub the outside of the chicken with garlic-infused olive oil.
3. Sprinkle salt and pepper on the chicken both inside and out.
4. Stuff the chicken with lemon quarters, rosemary, thyme, and parsley.
5. Place the chicken in a roasting pan and add the chicken broth to the bottom.
6. Roast in the preheated oven for about 1 hour and 30 minutes, or until the juices run clear when the thickest part of the thigh is pierced with a skewer.
7. Let the chicken sit for 10 minutes before cutting. Serve warm.

Prosciutto Wrapped Chicken

Ingredients:

- 4 boneless, skinless chicken breasts
- 8 slices of prosciutto
- 1 tablespoon garlic-infused olive oil
- 1 tablespoon fresh rosemary, chopped
- Salt and pepper to taste
- 1/2 cup low FODMAP chicken broth

Nutrition (per serving):

300 calories | 12g fat | 0g carbs | 45g protein | 0g sugar

Prep. time: 15 min   **Total time:** 40 min   **Servings:** 4

Directions:

1. Preheat your oven to 375°F (190°C).
2. Flatten the chicken breasts slightly with a meat mallet to ensure even cooking.
3. Season each chicken breast with some salt and pepper and sprinkle with chopped rosemary.
4. Use two slices of prosciutto to wrap around each chicken breast, covering the surface as much as possible.
5. Warm the garlic-infused olive oil in a large ovenproof skillet over medium-high heat.
6. Once hot, add the prosciutto-wrapped chicken breasts and sear for 2-3 minutes on each side or until the prosciutto is crispy.
7. Fill the skillet with the chicken broth and transfer the skillet to the oven.
8. Roast in the oven for about 15-20 minutes, or until the chicken is cooked through, about 165°F on the inside.
9. Serve the chicken breasts with some of the juices spooned over the top.

Balsamic Glazed Beef Ribs

Prep. time: 15 min   **Total time:** 3 hr 15 min   **Servings:** 4

Ingredients:

- 2 pounds beef ribs
- Salt and pepper to taste
- 2 tablespoons garlic-infused olive oil
- 1/2 cup balsamic vinegar
- 2 tablespoons brown sugar
- 1 tablespoon Dijon mustard (ensure it's low FODMAP)
- 1 teaspoon dried rosemary
- 1 teaspoon dried thyme

Nutrition (per serving):

500 calories | 35g fat | 10g carbs | 35g protein | 6g sugar

Directions:

1. Preheat your oven to 300°F (150°C).
2. Rub the beef ribs generously with salt and pepper on all sides.
3. In a large ovenproof skillet or Dutch oven, heat the garlic-infused olive oil over medium-high heat. Add the ribs and sear each side until browned, about 3-4 minutes per side.
4. In a small bowl, whisk together the Dijon mustard, balsamic vinegar, brown sugar, Dijon mustard, rosemary, and thyme to create the glaze.
5. Pour the glaze over the seared ribs, ensuring they are well coated.
6. Use the lid or aluminum foil to cover the skillet or Dutch oven, and then transfer to the preheated oven.
7. Braise the ribs in the oven until the meat is soft and falls off the bone for 2.5 to 3 hours. Baste occasionally with the cooking juices to keep the ribs moist.
8. Once cooked, remove the ribs from the oven and let them rest for a few minutes before serving.
9. Serve hot, drizzled with the reduced cooking juices and balsamic glaze from the pan.

Turkey Meatballs

Ingredients:

- 1 pound ground turkey
- 1/4 cup gluten-free breadcrumbs
- 1/4 cup grated Parmesan cheese
- 1 tablespoon garlic-infused olive oil
- 1 tablespoon fresh parsley, finely chopped
- 1 egg, beaten
- 1 teaspoon dried oregano
- Salt and pepper to taste
- 1/2 cup low FODMAP marinara sauce

Nutrition (per serving):

250 calories | 14g fat | 9g carbs | 23g protein | 2g sugar

Prep. time: 15 min **Total time:** 35 min **Servings:** 4

Directions:

1. Preheat your oven to 400°F (200°C). Line a baking sheet with parchment paper.
2. In a large bowl, combine the ground turkey, gluten-free breadcrumbs, grated Parmesan, garlic-infused olive oil, chopped parsley, beaten egg, dried oregano, salt, and pepper. Mix well to achieve an even distribution of all ingredients.
3. Shape the mixture into 1-inch balls and lay them on the prepared baking sheet.
4. Move them to the preheated oven and bake for 15-20 minutes, or until the meatballs are thoroughly cooked and slightly golden on the outside.
5. In a small saucepan, warm the low FODMAP marinara sauce over low heat.
6. Once the meatballs are cooked, add them to the saucepan and gently toss with the marinara sauce until well coated.
7. Serve the meatballs hot, garnished with extra chopped parsley.

Lemon Thyme Pork Tenderloin

Ingredients:

- 1 pork tenderloin (about 1 to 1.5 pounds)
- 2 tablespoons garlic-infused olive oil
- 2 tablespoons fresh thyme, finely chopped
- Zest of 1 lemon
- Juice of 1 lemon
- Salt and pepper to taste

Nutrition (per serving):

220 calories | 8g fat | 2g carbs | 32g protein | 1g sugar

Prep. time: 10 min **Total time:** 35 min **Servings:** 4

Directions:

1. Preheat your oven to 400°F (200°C).
2. Season dry pork tenderloin generously with salt and pepper.
3. In a small bowl, mix together the garlic-infused olive oil, chopped thyme, lemon zest, and lemon juice. Rub the mixture all over the pork tenderloin.
4. Place the pork in a roasting pan or on a rimmed baking sheet.
5. Roast the tenderloin in the preheated oven for 20-25 minutes, or until the thickest section registers 145°F (63°C) on a meat thermometer.
6. Take the pork out of the oven and give it five minutes to rest.
7. Slice the pork into medallions and serve right away.

Beef Stir Fry

Ingredients:

- 1 pound beef sirloin, thinly sliced
- 2 tablespoons garlic-infused olive oil
- 1 cup sliced carrots
- 1 cup sliced red bell pepper
- 1 cup chopped green beans
- 1/4 cup low FODMAP soy sauce (or tamari)
- 1 tablespoon ginger, peeled and grated
- 1 tablespoon sesame oil
- 2 tablespoons green onion tops (green parts only), sliced
- 1 teaspoon chili flakes (optional, adjust to taste)
- Salt and pepper to taste

Nutrition (per serving):

300 calories | 18g fat | 10g carbs | 25g protein | 4g sugar

Prep. time: 15 min **Total time:** 25 min **Servings:** 4

Directions:

1. Heat 1 tablespoon of garlic-infused olive oil in a big skillet or wok set over high heat.
2. Put the thinly sliced beef in the skillet and stir-fry for approximately 3-4 minutes until it turns brown. Take the meat out of the skillet and set it aside.
3. In the same skillet, add the remaining garlic-infused olive oil. Add the sliced carrots, red bell pepper, green beans, and stir-fry for about 5 minutes until the vegetables are tender but still crisp.
4. Return the beef to the skillet. Stir in the low FODMAP soy sauce, grated ginger, and sesame oil. Mix well to combine all the ingredients.
5. Cook for another 2 minutes to let the flavors blend.
6. Add salt and pepper to taste and chili flakes if desired.
7. Sprinkle with sliced green onion tops before serving.

Spiced Moroccan Chicken

Ingredients:

- 4 boneless, skinless chicken breasts
- 2 tablespoons garlic-infused olive oil
- 1 teaspoon ground cumin
- 1 teaspoon ground coriander
- 1 teaspoon ground cinnamon
- 1/2 teaspoon ground turmeric
- 1/2 teaspoon paprika
- Salt and pepper to taste
- 1 lemon, sliced for garnish
- Fresh cilantro, chopped

Nutrition (per serving):

260 calories | 9g fat | 3g carbs | 40g protein | 1g sugar

Prep. time: 20 min **Total time:** 50 min **Servings:** 4

Directions:

1. Mix coriander, salt, pepper, cumin, cinnamon, turmeric and paprika in a small bowl to create the spice rub.
2. Rub each chicken breast thoroughly with the spice mixture.
3. Heat the garlic-infused olive oil in a large skillet over medium heat.
4. Once hot, add the spiced chicken breasts to the skillet. Cook for about 5-7 minutes on each side or until the chicken is golden brown on the outside and thoroughly cooked.
5. Place the cooked chicken into a serving dish. Garnish with lemon slices and sprinkle with chopped fresh cilantro. Serve hot.

Maple-Glazed Chicken Breasts

Ingredients:

- 4 boneless, skinless chicken breasts
- Salt and pepper, to taste
- 2 tablespoons garlic-infused olive oil
- 1/4 cup pure maple syrup
- 2 tablespoons Dijon mustard (ensure low FODMAP)
- 1 tablespoon chopped fresh thyme
- 1 tablespoon chopped fresh rosemary
- Lemon wedges for serving

Nutrition (per serving):

295 calories | 10g fat | 14g carbs | 34g protein | 12g sugar

Prep. time: 10 min **Total time:** 30 min **Servings:** 4

Directions:

1. Preheat the oven to 375°F (190°C).
2. Season the chicken breasts using salt and pepper.
3. In a large oven-safe skillet, heat the garlic-infused olive oil over medium heat.
4. Add the chicken breasts to the skillet and cook on each side for 3 minutes, or until golden brown.
5. In a small bowl, combine the maple syrup, Dijon mustard, thyme, and rosemary.
6. Pour the maple mixture over the chicken in the skillet.
7. Move the skillet to the oven and bake for about 10-15 minutes, or until the chicken is thoroughly cooked and the glaze is caramelized.
8. Serve the chicken breasts with lemon wedges.

Spiced Chicken Drumettes

Ingredients:

- 2 pounds chicken drumettes
- 2 tablespoons garlic-infused olive oil
- 1 teaspoon smoked paprika
- 1 teaspoon ground cumin
- 1/2 teaspoon ground turmeric
- 1/2 teaspoon ground coriander
- 1/4 teaspoon cayenne pepper (optional)
- Salt and pepper, to taste
- Fresh cilantro, chopped (for garnish)
- Lemon wedges, for serving

Prep. time: 10 min **Total time:** 35 min **Servings:** 4

Directions:

1. Preheat the oven to 400°F (200°C).
2. Combine the garlic-infused olive oil, smoked paprika, cumin, turmeric, coriander, cayenne pepper, salt, and pepper in a large bowl.
3. Add the chicken drumettes to the bowl and mix to coat evenly with the spice mixture.
4. Arrange the coated drumettes on a baking sheet lined with parchment paper.
5. In a preheated oven, bake for 25 minutes or until the chicken is thoroughly cooked and the skin is crispy.
6. Add some chopped cilantro as a garnish, and serve with lemon wedges on the side.

Moroccan Spiced Lamb Ribs

Ingredients:

- 2 pounds lamb ribs
- Salt and pepper, to taste
- 2 tablespoons garlic-infused olive oil
- 1 teaspoon ground cumin
- 1 teaspoon smoked paprika
- 1 teaspoon ground coriander
- 1/2 teaspoon ground cinnamon
- 1/4 teaspoon cayenne pepper (optional)
- 1 tablespoon chopped fresh cilantro for garnish
- Lemon wedges for serving

Prep. time: 15 min   **Total time:** 2 hr 15 min   **Servings:** 4

Directions:

1. Preheat the oven to 325°F (160°C).
2. Season the lamb ribs with salt and pepper.
3. In a small bowl, combine the garlic-infused olive oil, cumin, smoked paprika, coriander, cinnamon, and cayenne pepper.
4. Evenly coat the lamb ribs with the spice mixture, rubbing it in.
5. Place the ribs on a baking sheet and cover with foil.
6. Bake for around 1 hour and 45 minutes in the preheated oven, or until the ribs are tender.
7. Remove the foil and set the oven to 400°F (200°C). Bake for 15 minutes more to crisp up the exterior.
8. Garnish with chopped cilantro and accompany with lemon wedges on the side.

Nutrition (per serving):

480 calories | 38g fat | 2g carbs | 32g protein | 0g sugar

Herbed Turkey Burgers

Ingredients:

- 1 pound ground turkey
- 1 tablespoon garlic-infused olive oil
- 1 tablespoon chopped fresh parsley
- 1 tablespoon chopped fresh chives
- 1 tablespoon chopped fresh basil
- Salt and pepper, to taste
- 4 gluten-free hamburger buns (optional, ensure low FODMAP)
- Lettuce leaves, for serving
- Tomato slices, for serving (if tolerated)

Prep. time: 10 min   **Total time:** 20 min   **Servings:** 4

Directions:

1. In a large bowl, mix together the ground turkey, garlic-infused olive oil, salt, pepper, parsley, chives and basil until well combined.
2. Shape 4 equal patties from the mixture.
3. Preheat a grill or grill pan over medium heat. Cook for about 5 minutes per side until the patties are thoroughly cooked and the internal temperature is 165°F (74°C).
4. Serve the turkey burgers on gluten-free hamburger buns if using, topped with lettuce leaves and tomato slices.

Nutrition (per serving):

210 calories | 12g fat | 1g carbs | 23g protein | 0g sugar

Beef and Fennel Casserole

Ingredients:

- 2 pounds beef chuck, cut into 1-inch cubes
- Salt and pepper, to taste
- 2 tablespoons garlic-infused olive oil
- 1 large fennel bulb, thinly sliced
- 1 cup diced carrots
- 1 cup low FODMAP beef broth
- 1/2 cup dry red wine
- 1 teaspoon dried thyme
- 1 teaspoon dried rosemary
- 2 bay leaves

Nutrition (per serving):

350 calories | 22g fat | 8g carbs | 24g protein | 3g sugar

Prep. time: 20 min **Total time:** 2 hr 20 min **Servings:** 6

Directions:

1. Preheat the oven to 325°F (160°C).
2. Add salt and pepper to the meat chunks for seasoning.
3. Place a large Dutch oven with garlic-infused oil over medium-high heat.
4. After adding the beef, cook it on all sides for eight to ten minutes. Remove the beef and set it aside.
5. Add the sliced fennel, carrots to the same pot and cook about 5 minutes until slightly tender.
6. Return the beef to the pot and add the beef broth, red wine, thyme, rosemary, and bay leaves.
7. After bringing it to a boil, cover and transfer it to the preheated oven.
8. Cook until the beef is soft for about 1 hour and 45 minutes.
9. Remove the bay leaves before serving.

Roasted Chicken with Fennel and Carrots

Ingredients:

- 4 chicken leg quarters
- Salt and pepper, to taste
- 2 tablespoons garlic-infused olive oil
- 1 large fennel bulb, cut into wedges
- 4 medium carrots, peeled and cut into sticks
- 1 teaspoon dried thyme
- 1 teaspoon dried rosemary
- Lemon wedges, for serving

Nutrition (per serving):

410 calories | 24g fat | 12g carbs | 35g protein | 5g sugar

Prep. time: 15 min **Total time:** 1 hr 15 min **Servings:** 4

Directions:

1. Preheat the oven to 400°F (200°C).
2. Sprinkle salt and pepper on the chicken leg quarters.
3. Place the chicken in a large roasting pan.
4. Toss the fennel wedges and carrot sticks with the garlic-infused olive oil, thyme, and rosemary.
5. Distribute the vegetables around the chicken in the roasting pan.
6. Roast in the oven for around 60 minutes, or until the chicken is golden and cooked through and the vegetables are tender.
7. Serve the chicken and vegetables hot, with lemon wedges on the side.

Pork Tenderloin with Oregano and Orange

Ingredients:

- 1 pork tenderloin (about 1.5 pounds)
- Salt and pepper, to taste
- 2 tablespoons garlic-infused olive oil
- 2 teaspoons dried oregano
- Zest of 1 orange
- 1/4 cup fresh orange juice
- 1 tablespoon Dijon mustard (ensure low FODMAP)
- 1 tablespoon white wine vinegar

Nutrition (per serving):

220 calories | 8g fat | 4g carbs | 32g protein | 2g sugar

Prep. time: 15 min **Total time:** 40 min **Servings:** 4

Directions:

1. Preheat the oven to 375°F (190°C).
2. Add oregano, salt, and pepper to the pork tenderloin to season it. In a large ovenproof skillet, heat the garlic-infused oil over medium-high heat.
3. Place the pork to the skillet and brown on all sides, about 6-8 minutes total.
4. In a small bowl, combine the orange juice, white wine vinegar, Dijon mustard, and orange zest.
5. Pour the orange mixture over the browned pork in the skillet.
6. Move the skillet to the preheated oven to roast the pork for 15-20 minutes or until a thermometer in the thickest part of the tenderloin reads 145°F (63°C).
7. Before slicing, give the pork five minutes to rest.
8. Serve the sliced pork drizzled with the cooking juices from the skillet.

Italian Meatloaf

Ingredients:

- 2 pounds ground beef
- 1/2 cup gluten-free breadcrumbs
- 1/4 cup lactose-free milk
- 2 tablespoons garlic-infused olive oil
- 1 tablespoon dried oregano
- 1 tablespoon dried basil
- 2 teaspoons salt
- 1 teaspoon ground black pepper
- 1/2 cup grated Parmesan cheese (ensure it's low lactose)
- 1 large egg
- 1/2 cup low FODMAP marinara sauce (for topping)

Prep. time: 20 min **Total time:** 1 hr 20 min **Servings:** 6

Directions:

1. Preheat the oven to 375°F (190°C).
2. Rub the outside of the chicken with garlic-infused olive oil.
3. Sprinkle salt and pepper on the chicken both inside and out.
4. Stuff the chicken with lemon quarters, rosemary, thyme, and parsley.
5. Place the chicken in a roasting pan and add the chicken broth to the bottom.
6. Roast in the preheated oven for about 1 hour and 30 minutes, or until the juices run clear when the thickest part of the thigh is pierced with a skewer.
7. Let the chicken sit for 10 minutes before cutting. Serve warm.

Beef Bolognese

Ingredients:

- 500g ground beef
- 2 tablespoons garlic-infused olive oil
- 1 large carrot, finely diced
- 1 stalk celery, finely diced
- 400g canned tomatoes, crushed
- 1/4 cup tomato paste
- 1 cup low FODMAP beef broth
- 1 teaspoon dried oregano
- 1 teaspoon dried basil
- 1 bay leaf
- Salt and pepper, to taste
- 1/2 cup grated Parmesan cheese (optional, for serving)
- Cooked gluten-free pasta (for serving)

Prep. time: 15 min | **Total time:** 60 min | **Servings:** 4

Directions:

1. In a large skillet, heat the garlic-infused olive oil over medium heat. After adding, sauté the ground beef, breaking it up with a spoon for 5 to 7 minutes until it is browned.
2. Add the celery and carrot to the skillet and cook for about 5 minutes until they begin to soften.
3. Stir in the beef broth, crushed tomatoes, tomato paste, oregano, basil, and bay leaf. Season with salt and pepper.
4. Let the mixture come to a boil, then decrease the heat and simmer uncovered for 30 minutes, stirring occasionally.
5. Take the bay leaf out and adjust the seasoning if needed.
6. Serve the Bolognese sauce over cooked gluten-free pasta and add grated Parmesan cheese on top if desired.

Nutrition (per serving):

380 calories | 20g fat | 15g carbs | 34g protein | 6g sugar

Grilled Tilapia with Oregano and Olive Oil

Ingredients:

- 4 tilapia fillets (6 oz each)
- 3 tablespoons olive oil
- 1 tablespoon dried oregano
- 1 tablespoon lemon juice
- 1/2 teaspoon salt
- 1/4 teaspoon freshly ground black pepper
- Lemon slices (for serving)

Prep. time: 5 min | **Total time:** 15 min | **Servings:** 4

Nutrition (per serving):

180 calories | 10g fat | 1g carbs | 23g protein | 0g sugar

Directions:

1. Preheat your grill to medium-high heat.
2. Mix lemon juice, olive oil, dried oregano, salt and black pepper in a small bowl.
3. Apply the oregano and olive oil mixture to both sides of each tilapia fillet.
4. Grill the fillets until the fish flakes easily with a fork for 4-5 minutes on each side.
5. Serve hot, garnished with lemon slices.

Spicy Grilled Tuna with Salsa

Ingredients:

- 4 tuna steaks (6 oz each)
- 1 tablespoon olive oil
- 1 teaspoon chili powder
- Salt and pepper, to tast

For the Salsa:

- 2 medium tomatoes, diced
- 1/2 cup cucumber, diced
- 1/4 cup red bell pepper, diced
- 1/4 cup fresh cilantro, chopped
- 2 tablespoons lime juice
- 1 tablespoon garlic-infused olive oil
- Salt and pepper, to taste

Prep. time: 15 min **Total time:** 21 min **Servings:** 4

Directions:

1. Preheat the grill to high heat.
2. Apply some olive oil to the tuna steaks and add pepper, salt, and chili powder for seasoning.
3. Grill the tuna steaks for about 3 minutes per side for medium-rare, or adjust the cooking time to your preferred doneness.
4. While the tuna grills, combine the tomatoes, cucumber, red bell pepper, cilantro, lime juice, and garlic-infused olive oil. Add salt and pepper and stir well to create the salsa.
5. Once the tuna is grilled, serve each steak with a generous portion of the fresh salsa on top.

Nutrition (per serving):

280 calories | 10g fat | 4g carbs | 40g protein | 2g sugar

Lemon Pepper Salmon

Ingredients:

- 4 salmon fillets (6 oz each)
- 2 tablespoons garlic-infused olive oil
- 2 teaspoons lemon zest
- 1 tablespoon lemon juice
- 1 teaspoon freshly ground black pepper
- 1/2 teaspoon salt
- 1 tablespoon chopped fresh parsley (for garnish)

Nutrition (per serving):

250 calories | 14g fat | 1g carbs | 30g protein | 0g sugar

Prep. time: 10 min **Total time:** 25 min **Servings:** 4

Directions:

1. Preheat your oven to 400°F (200°C). Line a baking sheet with parchment paper.
2. In a small bowl, mix the garlic-infused olive oil, lemon zest, lemon juice, black pepper, and salt.
3. Lay the salmon fillets out on the prepared baking sheet. Brush each fillet evenly with the lemon-pepper mixture.
4. Cook in the preheated oven until the salmon flakes with a fork for about 12-15 minutes.
5. Garnish with chopped fresh parsley before serving.

Seafood Paella

Prep. time: 15 min   **Total time:** 60 min   **Servings:** 4

Ingredients:

- 2 cups low FODMAP chicken broth
- A pinch of saffron threads
- 1 tablespoon garlic-infused olive oil
- 1 red bell pepper, thinly sliced
- 1/2 teaspoon smoked paprika
- 1 cup Arborio rice
- 200g large shrimp, peeled and deveined
- 200g scallops
- 200g firm white fish fillets, cut into chunks
- 1/4 cup chopped fresh parsley
- 1 lemon, cut into wedges
- Salt and pepper, to taste

Nutrition (per serving):

350 calories | 8g fat | 38g carbs | 28g protein | 3g sugar

Directions:

1. Warm the chicken broth and infuse it with saffron threads in a small saucepan. Keep it warm over low heat.
2. Heat the garlic-infused olive oil in a large skillet or paella pan over medium heat. Add the red bell pepper and sauté for about 5 minutes until soft.
3. Stir in the smoked paprika and Arborio rice, coating the rice in the oil and paprika for about 2 minutes.
4. Pour the warm saffron-infused broth over the rice, stir once, and then spread the rice evenly in the pan. Cook for around ten minutes on medium heat without stirring.
5. Arrange the shrimp, scallops, and fish chunks on the rice. Cover the pan with aluminum foil or with a lid and cook for 15 minutes more, or until the rice is tender and the seafood is cooked through.
6. Remove from heat and let it rest, covered, for about 5 minutes.
7. Add chopped parsley as a garnish and serve with lemon wedges on the side.

Cilantro Lime Shrimp

Prep. time: 10 min   **Total time:** 25 min   **Servings:** 4

Ingredients:

- 500g large shrimp, peeled and deveined
- 2 tablespoons garlic-infused olive oil
- 1/4 cup fresh cilantro, finely chopped
- 2 tablespoons lime juice
- 1 teaspoon lime zest
- 1/4 teaspoon red pepper flakes (optional)
- Salt and pepper, to taste

Nutrition (per serving):

150 calories | 7g fat | 1g carbs | 22g protein | 0g sugar

Directions:

1. In a large bowl, toss the shrimp with garlic-infused olive oil, salt, pepper, lime zest, lime juice, cilantro, and red pepper flakes (if using).
2. Heat a large skillet over medium-high heat.
3. Place the shrimp in the skillet in a single layer. Cook for 2-3 minutes on each side or until the shrimp turn pink and are cooked through.
4. Remove from heat and serve immediately. These can be enjoyed on their own or served over a bed of low FODMAP greens or rice.

Cod in Parsley Sauce

Ingredients:

- 4 cod fillets (6 oz each)
- Salt and pepper, to taste
- 2 tablespoons garlic-infused olive oil
- 2 tablespoons butter (or a low FODMAP alternative)
- 2 tablespoons gluten-free flour
- 1 cup low FODMAP vegetable broth
- 1/4 cup lactose-free cream
- 1/4 cup chopped fresh parsley
- Lemon wedges, for serving

Nutrition (per serving):

270 calories | 15g fat | 6g carbs | 28g protein | 1g sugar

Prep. time: 5 min **Total time:** 20 min **Servings:** 4

Directions:

1. Heat the garlic-infused olive oil in a large skillet over medium heat.
2. Sprinkle salt and pepper over the cod fillets.
3. Add the cod fillets to the skillet and cook on each side for 3-4 minutes, until the fish is well cooked and flakes with a fork. Take the cod out of the skillet and set it aside.
4. Melt the butter over medium heat using the same skillet. Stir in the gluten-free flour to form a roux, cooking for about 1 minute.
5. Gradually whisk in the vegetable broth and bring the mixture to a simmer. Cook until the sauce begins to thicken, three to five minutes.
6. Stir in the lactose-free cream and chopped parsley, add salt and pepper to taste.
7. Return the cod fillets to the skillet, spreading the sauce over them. Cook for another 2 minutes to heat the fish through.
8. Serve the cod fillets with the parsley sauce spooned over the top and lemon wedges on the side.

Sea Bass with Fennel and Tomatoes

Ingredients:

- 4 sea bass fillets (6 oz each)
- 2 tablespoons olive oil
- 1 large fennel bulb, thinly sliced
- 2 medium tomatoes, sliced
- 1 tablespoon fresh dill, chopped
- 1 lemon, sliced
- 1/2 teaspoon salt
- 1/4 teaspoon freshly ground black pepper

Nutrition (per serving):

200 calories | 10g fat | 6g carbs | 23g protein | 3g sugar

Prep. time: 10 min **Total time:** 30 min **Servings:** 4

Directions:

1. Preheat your oven to 375°F (190°C). Grease a baking dish with a little olive oil.
2. Arrange the sliced fennel and tomatoes in the bottom of the baking dish, and place the sea bass fillets on top.
3. Sprinkle salt and pepper on the fillets and drizzle with olive oil. Scatter lemon slices and fresh dill over the fish.
4. Cover the dish with aluminum foil and bake in the preheated oven for up to 20 minutes or until the fish is done and flakes with a fork.
5. Serve hot, ensuring each plate gets an even mix of vegetables and a fillet.

Prawn Stir Fry

Ingredients:

- 500g prawns, peeled and deveined
- 2 tablespoons garlic-infused olive oil
- 1 red bell pepper, thinly sliced
- 1 green bell pepper, thinly sliced
- 1 carrot, julienned
- 1 tablespoon ginger, finely grated
- 2 tablespoons soy sauce (gluten-free)
- 1 tablespoon sesame oil
- 1/4 teaspoon chili flakes
- 2 tablespoons green onion tops, for garnish

Prep. time: 20 min **Total time:** 50 min **Servings:** 4

Directions:

1. Heat the garlic-infused olive oil in a wok or a large skillet over medium-high heat.
2. Add the carrot and bell peppers to the skillet. Stir-fry until they start to soften, for about 5 minutes.
3. Add the prawns and ginger to the skillet. Continue to stir-fry until the prawns are pink and cooked through, about 3-4 minutes.
4. Stir in the sesame oil, soy sauce, and chili flakes if using, and cook for another minute to combine all the flavors.
5. Take off the heat and garnish with green onion tops before serving.

Nutrition (per serving):

210 calories | 10g fat | 6g carbs | 24g protein | 3g sugar

Grilled Scallops with Basil Dressing

Ingredients:

- 16 large scallops, cleaned
- 2 tablespoons olive oil
- Salt and pepper, to taste
- 1/4 cup fresh basil leaves, finely chopped
- 2 tablespoons lemon juice
- 1 teaspoon lemon zest
- 2 tablespoons garlic-infused olive oil
- Lemon wedges, for serving

Nutrition (per serving):

180 calories | 10g fat | 5g carbs | 20g protein | 1g sugar

Prep. time: 10 min **Total time:** 16 min **Servings:** 4

Directions:

1. Preheat your grill to high heat.
2. After patting the scallops dry with paper towels, coat the scallops with olive oil and season with salt and pepper.
3. In a small bowl, whisk together the chopped basil, lemon juice, lemon zest, and garlic-infused olive oil to make the dressing.
4. Grill the scallops on each side for 2-3 minutes until they have a nice sear and are opaque throughout.
5. Remove the scallops from the grill and arrange them on a serving platter. Drizzle the lemon basil dressing over the top.
6. Serve right away, accompanied by extra lemon wedges on the side.

Grilled Mackerel with Herb Salad

Ingredients:

- 4 whole mackerel, gutted and cleaned
- 2 tablespoons olive oil
- Salt and pepper, to taste
- 1 cup fresh parsley leaves
- 1 cup fresh mint leaves
- 1/4 cup chives, chopped
- 2 tablespoons lemon juice
- 1 tablespoon garlic-infused olive oil
- Lemon wedges, for serving

Prep. time: 10 min **Total time:** 20 min **Servings:** 4

Directions:

1. Preheat your grill to medium-high heat.
2. Rub each mackerel with olive oil and season both inside and out with salt and pepper.
3. Grill the mackerel for about 5 minutes on each side until the fish is cooked through and the skin is crispy.
4. Meanwhile, combine the parsley, mint, and chives in a large bowl to make the herb salad.
5. Dress the herb salad with lemon juice and garlic-infused olive oil, tossing gently to coat.
6. Serve the grilled mackerel with the fresh herb salad and lemon wedges on the side.

Nutrition (per serving):

310 calories | 21g fat | 1g carbs | 28g protein | 0g sugar

Fennel and Salmon Bake

Ingredients:

- 4 salmon fillets (6 oz each)
- 1 large fennel bulb, thinly sliced
- 2 tablespoons olive oil
- 1 lemon, thinly sliced
- 2 tablespoons fresh dill, chopped
- Salt and pepper, to taste

Prep. time: 15 min **Total time:** 1 hr 15 mins **Servings:** 4

Directions:

1. Preheat your oven to 400°F (200°C). Apply some olive oil to a baking dish.
2. Spread the sliced fennel evenly on the bottom of the baking dish.
3. Add one tablespoon of olive oil over the fennel and season with salt and pepper.
4. Place the salmon fillets on top of the fennel. After seasoning the salmon with salt and pepper, top each fillet with lemon slices and a sprinkle of chopped dill.
5. Spread the last tablespoon of olive oil over the salmon.
6. Bake for about 20 minutes in the preheated oven, or until the salmon is fully cooked and flakes easily with a fork. Serve hot.

Nutrition (per serving):

350 calories | 22g fat | 5g carbs | 34g protein | 0g sugar

Baked Trout with Dill and Lemon

Ingredients:

- 4 whole trout, gutted and cleaned
- 2 tablespoons olive oil
- Salt and pepper, to taste
- 1 lemon, thinly sliced
- 1/4 cup fresh dill, chopped
- Additional lemon wedges, for serving

Nutrition (per serving):

310 calories | 18g fat | 1g carbs | 34g protein | 0g sugar

Prep. time: 10 min   **Total time:** 25 min   **Servings:** 4

Directions:

1. Preheat your oven to 375°F (190°C). Line an oven tray with aluminum foil and lightly grease with olive oil.
2. Pat the trout dry with paper towels. Rub each trout inside and out with olive oil, then sprinkle inside and out with salt and pepper generously.
3. Stuff the cavity of each trout with lemon slices and a sprinkle of chopped dill.
4. Place the fish on the baking sheet and bake the trout for about 15 minutes in the preheated oven or until it is opaque and flakes easily with a fork.
5. Add a few more lemon wedges and some fresh dill as garnish. Serve hot.

Sesame Crusted Tuna Steak

Ingredients:

- 4 tuna steaks (6 oz each)
- 2 tablespoons sesame oil
- 1/4 cup sesame seeds
- Salt and pepper, to taste
- 2 tablespoons tamari sauce (gluten-free soy sauce)
- 1 tablespoon wasabi paste (check for FODMAP-friendly options)
- 1 tablespoon ginger, finely grated

Nutrition (per serving):

310 calories | 14g fat | 3g carbs | 40g protein | 1g sugar

Prep. time: 10 min   **Total time:** 16 mins   **Servings:** 4

Directions:

1. Preheat a skillet or a grill over medium-high heat.
2. Brush each tuna steak lightly with sesame oil and sprinkle salt and pepper on both sides.
3. Coat evenly on both sides of the tuna steaks with sesame seeds by pressing them firmly.
4. Grill the tuna steaks for around 3 minutes per side for medium-rare or longer for your preferred level of doneness.
5. In a small bowl, mix together the tamari sauce, wasabi paste, and grated ginger to create a dipping sauce.
6. Serve the sesame-crusted tuna steaks hot, accompanied by the wasabi dipping sauce.

Chapter 6: Cakes, Snacks and Desserts
Carrot Cake

Ingredients:

- 2 cups gluten-free all-purpose flour
- 3/4 cup granulated sugar
- 1/2 cup brown sugar
- 1 1/2 tsp baking powder
- 1/2 tsp baking soda
- 1/4 tsp salt
- 2 tsp cinnamon
- 1/2 cup vegetable oil
- 4 large eggs
- 2 cups grated carrots
- 1/2 cup chopped walnuts
- 1/4 cup unsweetened almond milk
- 1 tsp vanilla extract

Nutrition (per serving):

280 calories | 15g fat | 34g carbs | 5g protein | 20g sugar

Prep. time: 20 min   **Total time:** 50 min   **Servings:** 12

Directions

1. Preheat your oven to 350°F (175°C). Grease and flour a 9-inch round cake pan.
2. In a large bowl, mix together the flour, baking powder, baking soda, white sugar, brown sugar, salt and cinnamon.
3. In another bowl, blend the oil, eggs, almond milk, and vanilla extract until smooth.
4. Combine the wet and dry mixtures. Add the shredded carrots and chopped walnuts.
5. Transfer the batter to the prepared baking pan and level the surface with a spatula.
6. Bake in the preheated oven for about 30 minutes. A toothpick inserted in the center should come out clean.
7. Leave the cake in the pan for 10 minutes to cool, then shift it to a wire rack to cool completely.

Chocolate Pudding

Ingredients:

- 2 cups lactose-free milk
- 1/3 cup granulated sugar
- 1/4 cup cocoa powder, unsweetened
- 3 tablespoons cornstarch
- 1/4 teaspoon salt
- 1 teaspoon vanilla extract

Nutrition (per serving):

150 calories | 3g fat | 28g carbs | 4g protein | 17g sugar

Prep. time: 10 min   **Total time:** 20 min   **Servings:** 6

Directions:

1. Combine the cocoa powder, cornstarch, sugar, and salt in a medium saucepan.
2. Slowly add the milk into the saucepan, whisking continuously to ensure the mixture is smooth and free of lumps.
3. Put the saucepan on medium heat and stir the mixture constantly until it thickens and just begins to boil. Remove from heat immediately to prevent burning.
4. Stir in the vanilla extract.
5. Pour the pudding into serving dishes. Place plastic wrap directly on the surface of each pudding if you prefer skin not to form on top of the pudding.
6. Refrigerate for at least 2 hours until chilled and set.

Zucchini and Cheese Scones

Ingredients:

- 2 cups gluten-free all-purpose flour
- 1 tbsp baking powder
- 1/2 tsp salt
- 1/4 tsp black pepper
- 1/2 cup cold unsalted butter, cubed
- 1 cup grated zucchini (squeeze out excess moisture with a towel)
- 3/4 cup grated cheddar cheese (lactose-free if necessary)
- 2/3 cup lactose-free milk
- 1 large egg

Nutrition (per serving):

280 calories | 16g fat | 28g carbs | 8g protein | 2g sugar

Prep. time: 15 min **Total time:** 35 min **Servings:** 8

Directions:

1. Preheat your oven to 400°F (200°C). Prepare a baking sheet with parchment paper.
2. In a large bowl, whisk together the gluten-free flour, baking powder, salt, and black pepper.
3. Add the cold butter to the flour mixture rubbing it into the flour with your fingertips or a pastry blender until the coarse crumbs.
4. Stir in the grated zucchini and cheddar cheese.
5. In a small bowl, whisk together the lactose-free milk and egg. Add mixture to the dry ingredients, stirring just until the dough comes together.
6. Place the dough onto a surface lightly dusted with flour and shape it into a 1-inch thick circle. Use a sharp knife to cut the dough into 8 parts.
7. Transfer the wedges to the prepared baking sheet, spacing them slightly apart.
8. Bake in the preheated oven for about 20 minutes or until golden brown and cooked through.
9. Remove from the oven, let the scones cool slightly on the baking sheet, and transfer to a wire rack.
10. Enjoy warm. It can be stored in an airtight container for up to 2 days or frozen for longer.

Peanut Butter Cookies

Ingredients:

- 1 cup natural peanut butter (sugar-free, without additives)
- 1 cup granulated sugar
- 1 large egg
- 1 tsp baking soda
- 1/2 tsp vanilla extract

Nutrition (per serving):

410 calories | 24g fat | 12g carbs | 35g protein | 5g sugar

Prep. time: 10 min   **Total time:** 20 min   **Servings:** 24

Directions:

1. Preheat your oven to 350°F (175°C). Prepare a baking sheet with parchment paper.
2. In a bowl, combine peanut butter, sugar, egg, baking soda, and vanilla extract. Mix until all the ingredients are well combined, and the mixture is smooth.
3. Take tablespoon-sized portions of dough and shape them into balls. Transfer the dough balls to the prepared baking sheet, spacing them about 2 inches apart.
4. Use a fork to gently press down on each dough ball, creating a criss-cross pattern.
5. Bake in the preheated oven for 10 minutes or until the edges are slightly golden. Be careful not to overbake.
6. After taking the cookies out of the oven, let them sit on the baking sheet for 5 minutes, and afterward, transfer them to a wire rack to cool down completely.

Almond Joy Bars

Ingredients:

- 2 cups shredded coconut, unsweetened
- 1/3 cup coconut oil, melted
- 1/3 cup maple syrup
- 1 tsp vanilla extract
- 16 whole almonds
- 1/2 cup dark chocolate chips (low FODMAP friendly, lactose-free)

Nutrition (per serving):

220 calories | 18g fat | 15g carbs | 2g protein | 10g sugar

Prep. time: 15 min   **Total time:** 15 min   **Servings:** 16

Directions:

1. In a mixing bowl, combine well-shredded coconut, maple syrup, coconut oil, and vanilla extract.
2. Prepare a baking pan (8x8 inches), lining it with parchment paper.
3. Use your hands or a spatula to press the coconut mixture into the pan firmly. Distribute almonds on top evenly.
4. Use a small microwave-safe bowl to melt the chocolate chips, microwaving in 30-second intervals. Stir after each interval until smooth.
5. Drizzle the melted chocolate over the coconut and almonds.
6. Refrigerate the pan for at least 2 hours until the mixture is firm.
7. Once set, lift the mixture out of the pan, holding the edges of the parchment paper by hands and cut into 16 bars.

Lemon Cupcakes

Ingredients:

- 1 1/2 cups gluten-free all-purpose flour
- 3/4 cup granulated sugar
- 1/2 tsp baking powder
- 1/4 tsp baking soda
- 1/4 tsp salt
- 1/2 cup unsalted butter, softened
- 2 large eggs
- 1/4 cup lactose-free sour cream
- 1/4 cup lactose-free milk
- 2 tbsp lemon zest
- 1/4 cup fresh lemon juice
- 1 tsp vanilla extract

Nutrition (per serving):

180 calories | 9g fat | 23g carbs | 3g protein | 12g sugar

Prep. time: 15 min   **Total time:** 35 min   **Servings:** 12

Directions:

1. Preheat your oven to 350°F (175°C). Prepare a muffin tin with cupcake liners.
2. In a bowl, mix the gluten-free flour with baking soda, baking powder and salt.
3. In another large bowl, blend the butter and sugar until the mixture is light and creamy. Beat in the eggs one at a time.
4. Stir the lemon juice, lemon zest, and vanilla extract into the mixture.
5. Alternately, add the mixture of flour and lactose-free milk with sour cream to the butter mixture, starting and ending with the flour mixture. Mix until just combined.
6. Spread the batter evenly among the lined muffin cups, filling each about two-thirds full.
7. Bake for about 20 minutes or until a toothpick placed in a cupcake center comes out clean.
8. Keep the cupcakes in the pan for 5 minutes, then transfer them to a wire rack to cool completely.

Pumpkin Pie

Ingredients:

- 1 9-inch gluten-free pie crust
- 2 cups pumpkin puree (make sure it's pure pumpkin)
- 3/4 cup lactose-free heavy cream
- 1/2 cup maple syrup
- 3 large eggs
- 1 tsp ground cinnamon
- 1/2 tsp ground ginger
- 1/4 tsp ground nutmeg
- 1/4 tsp salt

Nutrition (per serving):

280 calories | 15g fat | 35g carbs | 5g protein | 16g sugar

Prep. time: 15 min   **Total time:** 60 min   **Servings:** 8

Directions:

1. Preheat your oven to 375°F (190°C).
2. In a large mixing bowl, combine the pumpkin puree, lactose-free heavy cream, maple syrup, eggs, cinnamon, ginger, nutmeg, and salt. Whisk together until well blended.
3. Pour the pumpkin mixture into the gluten-free pie crust.
4. Put the pie on a baking sheet and bake it in the preheated oven for 45 minutes, or until the filling is set and the crust is golden.
5. Take the pie out of the oven and leave it on a wire rack for at least 2 hours before serving to allow the filling to firm up.

Oatmeal Raisin Cookies

Prep. time: 15 min   **Total time:** 25 min   **Servings:** 24

Ingredients:

- 1 1/2 cups gluten-free oats
- 1 cup gluten-free all-purpose flour
- 1/2 tsp baking soda
- 1/2 tsp salt
- 1 tsp cinnamon
- 1/2 cup unsalted butter, softened
- 1/2 cup granulated sugar
- 1/4 cup brown sugar
- 2 large eggs
- 1 tsp vanilla extract
- 3/4 cup raisins

Nutrition (per serving):

130 calories | 6g fat | 18g carbs | 2g protein | 10g sugar

Directions:

1. Preheat your oven to 350°F (175°C). Prepare a baking sheet with parchment paper.
2. Mix oats, flour, baking soda, salt, and cinnamon in a small bowl.
3. In a bigger bowl, blend the butter, granulated and brown sugar until the mixture is light and creamy.
4. Beat the eggs into the mixture one at a time, then mix in the vanilla extract.
5. Gradually stir the dry components into the wet ingredients until just mixed. Fold in the raisins.
6. Place a full tablespoon portions of the dough onto the prepared baking sheet with a space of 2 inches in between.
7. Bake for 10 minutes or until the edges turn golden brown.
8. After removing the cookies from the oven, let them rest on the baking sheet for several minutes before placing them to a wire rack to cool completely.

Sesame Rice Cakes

Prep. time: 10 min   **Total time:** 30 min   **Servings:** 8

Ingredients:

- 2 cups cooked jasmine rice (cooled)
- 1/4 cup sesame seeds
- 2 eggs
- 1/4 cup green onions, green parts only, finely chopped
- 1/4 tsp salt
- 2 tbsp gluten-free tamari sauce
- 1/4 cup sesame oil (for frying)

Nutrition (per serving):

180 calories | 14g fat | 12g carbs | 4g protein | 1g sugar

Directions:

1. In a large bowl, mix the cooked jasmine rice, sesame seeds, eggs, chopped green onions, salt, and tamari sauce until well combined.
2. Pour sesame oil into a large skillet and warm over medium heat.
3. Form the rice mixture into small patties, each about 3 inches in diameter.
4. Fry the patties in the hot oil for 3-4 minutes on each side or until golden brown and crispy.
5. Remove the rice cakes from the skillet and use paper towels to drain any extra oil.
6. Serve warm.

Orange Polenta Cake

Ingredients:

- 1 cup fine polenta
- 1/2 cup gluten-free all-purpose flour
- 2 tsp baking powder
- 1/2 tsp salt
- 3/4 cup unsalted butter, softened
- 1 cup granulated sugar
- 3 large eggs
- 2 tsp orange zest
- 1/4 cup fresh orange juice
- 1 tsp vanilla extract
- Powdered sugar for dusting (optional)

Nutrition (per serving):

280 calories | 15g fat | 35g carbs | 4g protein | 20g sugar

Prep. time: 15 min **Total time:** 55 min **Servings:** 10

Directions:

1. Preheat your oven to 350°F (175°C). Prepare an 8-inch round cake pan greasing it and lining with parchment paper.
2. In a bowl, whisk together polenta, gluten-free flour, baking powder, and salt.
3. Cream the butter and sugar together in a big bowl until fluffy and light. Beat in the eggs, one at a time, until well combined.
4. Add the vanilla extract, orange zest, and orange juice and stir.
5. Stir the dry components into the wet ingredients gradually until combined.
6. Spread the batter in the prepared pan and smooth the top with a spatula.
7. The cake is ready in about 40 minutes when a toothpick inserted into the middle comes out clean.
8. Let the cake rest in the pan for 10 minutes, then turn it out onto a wire rack and let cool completely.
9. Before serving, dust with powdered sugar, if desired.

Oat and Peanut Butter Energy Balls

Ingredients:

- 1 cup gluten-free oats
- 1/2 cup natural peanut butter (sugar-free and without additives)
- 1/4 cup maple syrup
- 1/4 cup mini dark chocolate chips (lactose-free if necessary)
- 1/4 cup chia seeds
- 1 tsp vanilla extract

Nutrition (per serving):

150 calories | 8g fat | 17g carbs | 5g protein | 6g sugar

Prep. time: 15 min **Total time:** 15 min **Servings:** 12

Directions:

1. In a large bowl, combine all ingredients: oats, peanut butter, maple syrup, chocolate chips, chia seeds, and vanilla extract.
2. Stir the mixture until everything is well combined.
3. The texture should be sticky and hold together when pressed.
4. Roll the mixture into small walnut-sized balls using your hands.
5. Transfer the balls to a parchment-lined baking sheet and refrigerate for at least 1 hour to set.
6. Once set, the energy balls can be kept in an airtight container in the fridge for up to one week or in the freezer for longer storage.

Chocolate Cake

Ingredients:

- 1 3/4 cups gluten-free all-purpose flour
- 3/4 cup unsweetened cocoa powder
- 2 cups granulated sugar
- 1 1/2 tsp baking powder
- 1 1/2 tsp baking soda
- 1 tsp salt
- 2 large eggs
- 1 cup lactose-free milk
- 1/2 cup vegetable oil
- 2 tsp vanilla extract
- 1 cup boiling water

Nutrition (per serving):

320 calories | 12g fat | 50g carbs | 4g protein | 30g sugar

Prep. time: 15 min   **Total time:** 50 min   **Servings:** 12

Directions:

1. Preheat your oven to 350°F (175°C). Grease and flour two 9-inch round cake pans.
2. In a large bowl, sift together the flour, cocoa powder, baking powder, baking soda, add sugar and salt.
3. Add the eggs, lactose-free milk, oil and vanilla extract to the flour mixture and combine well.
4. Stir in the boiling water to get a thin batter.
5. Distribute the batter between the prepared pans.
6. Bake until a toothpick inserted into the center of the cake comes out clean for 30 to 35 minutes.
7. Let the cakes rest in the pans for 10 minutes, then take them out onto a wire rack to cool completely.

Coconut Rice Pudding

Ingredients:

- 1 cup jasmine rice
- 1 can (13.5 oz) coconut milk (full-fat)
- 2 cups lactose-free milk
- 1/3 cup granulated sugar
- 1/4 tsp salt
- 1 tsp vanilla extract
- Toasted coconut flakes, ground cinnamon for garnish

Nutrition (per serving):

310 calories | 14g fat | 42g carbs | 6g protein | 12g sugar

Prep. time: 5 min   **Total time:** 30 min   **Servings:** 6

Directions:

1. Rinse the jasmine rice several times under cold water until the water runs clean.
2. In a big saucepan, combine the rinsed rice with coconut milk, lactose-free milk, sugar, and salt.
3. Simmer the mixture uncovered over low heat after bringing it to a boil. Cook, stirring occasionally, for around 20–25 minutes, until the mixture thickens and the rice is soft.
4. Take off the heat and stir in the vanilla extract.
5. Serve warm or let cool, then chill in the refrigerator to serve cold. If desired, garnish with toasted coconut flakes and a sprinkle of ground cinnamon for added flavor.

Gluten-Free Pumpkin Bread

Prep. time: 15 min   **Total time:** 1 hr 5 min   **Servings:** 12

Ingredients:

- 1 3/4 cups gluten-free all-purpose flour
- 1 tsp baking soda
- 1/2 tsp salt
- 1 1/2 tsp cinnamon
- 1/2 tsp nutmeg
- 1/4 tsp cloves
- 1/4 tsp ginger
- 1 cup pumpkin puree (not pie filling)
- 1 cup granulated sugar
- 1/2 cup vegetable oil
- 1/4 cup lactose-free yogurt
- 2 large eggs
- 1 tsp vanilla extract
- Optional: 1/2 cup walnuts or pecans

Directions:

1. Preheat your oven to 350°F (175°C). Grease and flour a 9x5 inch loaf pan.
2. In a large bowl, whisk together the gluten-free flour, baking soda, salt, cinnamon, nutmeg, cloves, and ginger.
3. In another bowl, combine the pumpkin puree, lactose-free yogurt, eggs, sugar, vegetable oil and vanilla extract until smooth.
4. Gradually stir the dry components into the wet ingredients until just combined. Fold in nuts if using.
5. Prepare the loaf pan and transfer the batter into it, smoothing the top.
6. Bake the bread in the preheated oven for 50 minutes until a toothpick inserted into the center comes out clean.
7. After 10 minutes of resting in the pan, take the bread out to a wire rack to cool completely.

Nutrition (per serving):

230 calories | 11g fat | 32g carbs | 3g protein | 16g sugar

Cheese Crackers

Prep. time: 15 min   **Total time:** 30 min   **Servings:** 4

Ingredients:

- 1 cup gluten-free all-purpose flour
- 1/2 tsp salt
- 1/2 tsp paprika
- 1/4 tsp garlic powder (optional, omit if sensitive to garlic)
- 4 tbsp cold unsalted butter, cut into small pieces
- 1 cup grated cheddar cheese (lactose-free if necessary)
- 2-3 tbsp cold water

Nutrition (per serving):

350 calories | 25g fat | 25g carbs | 10g protein | 1g sugar

Directions:

1. Preheat your oven to 375°F (190°C). Line a baking sheet with parchment paper.
2. Combine flour, garlic powder, paprika and salt in a large bowl. Add the butter and incorporate it into the flour mixture with your fingers or a pastry cutter until it resembles coarse crumbs.
3. Stir in the grated cheese. Slowly add cold water, one tablespoon at a time, mixing until the dough sticks into a ball.
4. Roll the dough until 1/8 inch thick between two parchment paper sheets.
5. Remove the top layer of parchment. Cut the dough into small triangles, squares or other desired shapes with a knife.
6. Move the shapes to the prepared baking sheet. If desired, use a fork to prick each cracker several times.
7. Bake for about 15 minutes or until the edges are just starting to brown.
8. Take the crackers out of the oven and leave them on the baking sheet for 5 minutes, then place on a wire rack until cool completely.

Sweet Potato Brownies

Prep. time: 15 min   **Total time:** 40 min   **Servings:** 12

Ingredients:

- 1 cup mashed sweet potato (around 1 large sweet potato)
- 1/2 cup natural peanut butter (use almond butter for a different flavor)
- 1/4 cup cocoa powder
- 1/2 cup maple syrup
- 1/2 tsp baking soda
- Optional: 1/2 cup dark chocolate chips (lactose-free)

Nutrition (per serving):

180 calories | 10g fat | 20g carbs | 4g protein | 12g sugar

Directions:

1. Preheat your oven to 350°F (175°C). Line with parchment paper or grease 8x8 inch baking pan.
2. Combine the mashed sweet potato, peanut butter, cocoa powder, maple syrup, and baking soda in a large bowl. Mix until smooth and well combined.
3. If using, fold in the chocolate chips.
4. Fill the baking pan with the mixture and spread evenly.
5. Bake for 25 minutes, or until the center is set and the edges are firm.
7. Let the brownies cool in the pan for at least 10 minutes before cutting into squares.

Cheddar and Herb Muffins

Ingredients:

- 2 cups gluten-free all-purpose flour
- 1 tbsp baking powder
- 1/2 tsp salt
- 1/2 tsp pepper
- 1 tbsp dried herbs (such as chives and parsley or Italian seasoning)
- 1 cup grated cheddar cheese (lactose-free if necessary)
- 1 cup lactose-free milk
- 1/4 cup vegetable oil
- 2 large eggs

Nutrition (per serving):

200 calories | 10g fat | 22g carbs | 6g protein | 2g sugar

Prep. time: 15 min **Total time:** 35 min **Servings:** 12

Directions:

1. Preheat your oven to 375°F (190°C). Grease the muffin cups or line a tin with paper liners.
2. In a large bowl, whisk together the gluten-free flour, baking powder, salt, dried herbs and pepper.
3. Stir in the grated cheddar cheese.
4. In another bowl, whisk together the lactose-free milk, vegetable oil, and eggs.
5. Add the wet ingredients to the dry ingredients, stirring until combined (do not overmix).
6. Fill about two-thirds of each muffin cup with the batter.
7. Bake in the preheated oven until the tops are brown, for approximately 20 minutes, checking with a toothpick inserted into the center of a muffin to ensure it comes out clean.
8. Allow the muffins to sit in the cups for 5 minutes, and move them to a wire rack to cool completely.

Almond Banana Muffins

Ingredients:

- 2 medium ripe bananas, mashed
- 3/4 cup almond flour
- 1/4 cup coconut flour
- 1/2 cup lactose-free yogurt
- 2 large eggs
- 1/4 cup maple syrup
- 1 teaspoon baking powder
- 1/2 teaspoon baking soda
- 1/4 teaspoon salt
- 1 teaspoon vanilla extract
- 1/2 cup chopped walnuts (optional)

Nutrition (per serving):

150 calories | 9g fat | 17g carbs | 5g protein | 8g sugar

Prep. time: 15 min **Total time:** 35 min **Servings:** 12

Directions:

1. Preheat your oven to 350°F (175°C). Use paper liners in a muffin tin or grease it with a bit of coconut oil.
2. Combine the mashed bananas, almond flour, coconut flour, lactose-free yogurt, eggs, maple syrup, baking powder, baking soda, salt, and vanilla extract in a large bowl. Mix well until the batter is smooth and all ingredients are evenly incorporated.
3. Fold in the chopped walnuts if using.
4. Spread the batter evenly among the 12 muffin cups, filling each about 2/3 full.
5. Bake the muffins for about 20 minutes or until a toothpick inserted in the middle comes out clean.
6. Take the muffins out of the oven and let them cool in the pan for 5 minutes, then move to a wire rack for further cooling.

Baked Oatmeal Cups

Ingredients:

- 3 cups gluten-free oats
- 1 tsp baking powder
- 1/2 tsp salt
- 1 tsp cinnamon
- 2 large eggs
- 1 cup lactose-free milk
- 1/2 cup maple syrup
- 1/4 cup vegetable oil
- 1 tsp vanilla extract
- 1 cup mixed low-FODMAP fruits (such as blueberries, strawberries, and chopped oranges)

Nutrition (per serving):

180 calories | 7g fat | 27g carbs | 4g protein | 9g sugar

Prep. time: 10 min   **Total time:** 30 min   **Servings:** 12

Directions:

1. Preheat your oven to 375°F (190°C). Grease a 12-cup muffin tin or use paper liners.
2. Mix the oats, cinnamon, baking powder, and salt in a big bowl.
3. Beat the eggs, lactose-free milk, maple syrup, vegetable oil and vanilla extract in a separate bowl.
4. Add the wet ingredients to the dry components and mix until combined.
5. Gently fold in the mixed fruits.
6. Spread the mixture among the muffin cups evenly, filling each about three-quarters full.
7. Place in the preheated oven and bake for 20 minutes, or until the tops turn golden and a toothpick inserted into the center of a muffin comes out clean.
8. Let the oatmeal cups stay in the pan for 5 minutes, then transfer them to a wire rack to cool completely.

Chapter 7: Condiments
Garlic-Infused Olive Oil

Ingredients:
- 1 cup extra virgin olive oil
- 3 cloves garlic, whole

Nutrition (per serving):
120 calories | 14g fat | 0g carbs | 0g protein | 0g sugar

Prep. time: 5 min   **Total time:** 50 min   **Servings:** 1 cup

Directions:
1. To release the flavors, peel and lightly smash the garlic cloves, ensuring they remain intact to facilitate easy removal later.
2. Add the garlic cloves along with the olive oil to a small saucepan. Heat the mixture over low heat for about 10 minutes until it begins to bubble gently around the garlic. Be cautious not to let the garlic brown or burn.
3. Decrease the heat to the lowest setting and let the oil infuse for about 35 minutes. Monitor the heat closely to ensure the oil does not overheat, or start frying the garlic.
4. After 35 minutes, remove the pan from the heat and let the oil cool completely.
5. Strain the oil through a cheesecloth or a fine sieve to remove all pieces of garlic. Bottle the infused oil and store it in a cool, dark place.

Lemon Tahini Dressing

Ingredients:
- 1/2 cup tahini (sesame seed paste)
- 1/4 cup lemon juice, freshly squeezed
- 1/4 cup water, more as needed to thin
- 2 tablespoons garlic-infused olive oil
- 1 tablespoon maple syrup (optional for a slight sweetness)
- 1/4 teaspoon salt, or to taste

Nutrition (per serving):
98 calories | 9g fat | 3g carbs | 2g protein | 1g sugar

Prep. time: 10 min   **Total time:** 10 min   **Servings:** 1 cup

Directions:
1. In a medium bowl, mix the tahini and lemon juice well. Stir until the mixture thickens and becomes slightly stiff.
2. Gradually add the water, stirring continuously. The dressing will initially become thicker. Continue to add water until it reaches your desired consistency.
3. Stir in the garlic-infused olive oil, maple syrup (if using), and salt. Whisk until all ingredients are well combined, and the dressing is smooth and creamy.
4. Taste and adjust the seasoning, adding more salt or lemon juice if needed.
5. Transfer to a jar or container and store in the refrigerator for up to one week. Shake or stir before using if separation occurs.

Pesto

Ingredients:

- 2 cups fresh basil leaves, packed
- 1/3 cup pine nuts or walnuts
- 1/2 cup grated Parmesan cheese
- 1/3 cup garlic-infused olive oil
- 1 tablespoon lemon juice
- Salt, to taste

Nutrition (per serving):

190 calories | 19g fat | 2g carbs | 4g protein | 0g sugar

Prep. time: 10 min **Total time:** 10 min **Servings:** 1 cup

Directions:

1. Combine the pine nuts and basil leaves in a food processor. Pulse a few times until coarsely chopped.
2. Blend once more after adding the grated Parmesan cheese.
3. Slowly add the lemon juice and garlic-infused olive oil while the processor runs. Continue processing until the mixture becomes creamy and smooth.
4. Add salt to taste, then pulse again to mix.
5. Spoon the pesto into a container or a jar. If not using immediately, lightly coat the surface with olive oil to stop oxidation. Store in the refrigerator for up to one week or freeze for longer storage.

Barbecue Sauce

Ingredients:

- 1 cup tomato sauce (ensure no garlic or onion is added)
- 1/4 cup pure maple syrup
- 1/4 cup apple cider vinegar
- 2 tablespoons dark brown sugar
- 2 tablespoons Worcestershire sauce (ensure gluten-free and onion/garlic-free)
- 1 tablespoon smoked paprika
- 1 teaspoon mustard powder
- 1/2 teaspoon salt
- 1/2 teaspoon black pepper
- 1/4 teaspoon cayenne pepper (optional, adjust to taste)

Prep. time: 20 min **Total time:** 35 min **Servings:** 2 cups

Directions:

1. In a medium saucepan, combine tomato sauce, maple syrup, apple cider vinegar, brown sugar, Worcestershire sauce, smoked paprika, mustard powder, salt, cayenne pepper and black pepper.
2. Bring the mixture to a simmer over medium heat, stirring frequently to ensure the ingredients are well combined.
3. Decrease the heat to low and simmer until the sauce thickens to your desired consistency, about 20 minutes. Stir occasionally to prevent sticking or burning.
4. Taste and adjust the seasoning, adding extra pepper, salt or cayenne for heat if desired.
5. Take the sauce off the stove and let it cool. Refrigerate after transferring to a jar or other container until needed. The sauce can be kept in the refrigerator for up to 2 weeks.

Cucumber Dill Yogurt Dip

Ingredients:

- 1 cup lactose-free Greek yogurt
- 1/2 cup cucumber, finely grated and excess moisture squeezed out
- 2 tablespoons fresh dill, finely chopped
- 1 tablespoon lemon juice
- 1 tablespoon garlic-infused olive oil
- 1/4 teaspoon salt, or to taste
- 1/8 teaspoon black pepper, or to taste

Prep. time: 10 min   **Total time:** 10 min   **Servings:** 1 cup

Directions:

1. In a medium bowl, combine the lactose-free Greek yogurt, grated cucumber, chopped dill, lemon juice, and garlic-infused olive oil.
2. Blend all the ingredients thoroughly, and season with salt and pepper to taste.
3. Cover the bowl with plastic wrap and chill it for at least 1 hour to let the tastes merge together.
4. Before serving, stir the dip well to mix any liquid that may have separated. Serve chilled with your choice of low FODMAP veggies or chips.

Nutrition (per serving):

35 calories | 2g fat | 3g carbs | 2g protein | 2g sugar

Green Onion Aioli

Ingredients:

- 1 cup mayonnaise (ensure it's low FODMAP, without garlic or onion)
- 1/4 cup green onion tops, finely chopped (green parts only)
- 2 tablespoons lemon juice
- 1 tablespoon Dijon mustard
- 1/2 teaspoon salt
- 1/4 teaspoon black pepper

Prep. time: 10 min   **Total time:** 10 min   **Servings:** 1 cup

Directions:

1. In a medium bowl, combine the mayonnaise, finely chopped green onion tops, lemon juice, and Dijon mustard.
2. Stir thoroughly until all ingredients are well incorporated. Season with salt and pepper.
3. Transfer the aioli to a jar or container with a lid and refrigerate for at least 30 minutes to let the flavors merge.
4. Serve the cold aioli as a sandwich spread, as a dip for veggies, or as a condiment for grilled meats and fish.

Nutrition (per serving):

100 calories | 10g fat | 0.5g carbs | 0g protein | 0g sugar

Italian Dressing

Ingredients:

- 3/4 cup extra virgin olive oil
- 1/4 cup red wine vinegar
- 2 tablespoons lemon juice
- 1 teaspoon Dijon mustard
- 1 teaspoon dried oregano
- 1 teaspoon dried basil
- 1/2 teaspoon salt
- 1/4 teaspoon black pepper
- 1/4 teaspoon dried thyme
- 1 tablespoon garlic-infused olive oil

Prep. time: 10 min | **Total time:** 10 min | **Servings:** 1 cup

Directions:

1. In a small bowl or jar, combine the extra virgin olive oil, red wine vinegar, lemon juice, Dijon mustard, dried oregano, dried basil, salt, black pepper, dried thyme, and garlic-infused olive oil.
2. Whisk or shake the container vigorously until all ingredients are well blended, and the dressing is emulsified.
3. Adjust the seasoning with salt and pepper or herbs according to your preference.
4. Store the dressing refrigerated in a sealed container. Shake well before each use. The dressing should keep well for up to 2 weeks.

Nutrition (per serving):

120 calories | 13g fat | 0.5g carbs | 0g protein | 0g sugar

Tzatziki Sauce

Ingredients:

- 1 cup lactose-free Greek yogurt
- 1/2 cup cucumber, finely grated, excess moisture squeezed out
- 1 tablespoon dill, finely chopped
- 1 tablespoon lemon juice
- 1 tablespoon garlic-infused olive oil
- 1/4 teaspoon salt, or to taste
- 1/8 teaspoon black pepper

Prep. time: 15 min | **Total time:** 15 min | **Servings:** 1 cup

Directions:

1. In a medium bowl, combine the lactose-free Greek yogurt, finely grated cucumber, chopped dill, lemon juice, and garlic-infused olive oil.
2. Mix all the ingredients until well combined. Season with salt and pepper to taste.
3. Refrigerate in a covered bowl for at least 1 hour to let the flavors merge.
4. Before serving, stir the sauce again to ensure it is well-mixed. Adjust seasoning if necessary. Serve chilled as a dip for vegetables, with grilled meats, or as a refreshing condiment for wraps and sandwiches.

Nutrition (per serving):

45 calories | 3g fat | 3g carbs | 2g protein | 2g sugar

Hummus

Prep. time: 10 min   **Total time:** 50 min   **Servings:** 2 cups

Ingredients:

- 1 cup canned chickpeas, rinsed and drained
- 1/4 cup tahini (sesame seed paste)
- 1/4 cup lemon juice
- 1/4 cup water, more as needed for consistency
- 1/3 cup garlic-infused olive oil
- 1/2 teaspoon salt, or to taste
- 1/4 teaspoon ground cumin
- Paprika, for garnish (optional)

Directions:

1. Combine chickpeas, tahini, lemon juice, water, and half of the garlic-infused olive oil in a food processor. Blend until smooth.
2. While blending, gradually add the remaining garlic-infused olive oil until the hummus reaches your desired creamy consistency.
3. Season with salt and cumin. Blend again to mix thoroughly.
4. Transfer the hummus to a serving bowl. Drizzle with some extra garlic-infused olive oil and sprinkle with paprika if desired.
5. Serve with low FODMAP vegetables or gluten-free pita chips for dipping.

Nutrition (per serving):

100 calories | 8g fat | 6g carbs | 3g protein | 1g sugar

Cranberry Sauce

Prep. time: 5 min   **Total time:** 15 min   **Servings:** 1 cup

Ingredients:

- 2 cups fresh or frozen cranberries
- 1/2 cup water
- 1/2 cup pure maple syrup
- 1 teaspoon orange zest (optional)
- 1 cinnamon stick (optional)

Directions:

1. In a medium bowl, combine the lactose-free Greek yogurt, finely grated cucumber, chopped dill, lemon juice, and garlic-infused olive oil.
2. Mix all the ingredients until well combined. Season with salt and pepper to taste.
3. Refrigerate in a covered bowl for at least 1 hour to let the flavors merge.
4. Before serving, stir the sauce again to ensure it is well-mixed. Adjust seasoning if necessary. Serve chilled as a dip for vegetables, with grilled meats, or as a refreshing condiment for wraps and sandwiches.

Nutrition (per serving):

70 calories | 0g fat | 18g carbs | 0g protein | 12g sugar

Mint Yogurt Sauce

Ingredients:

- 1 cup lactose-free Greek yogurt
- 1/4 cup fresh mint leaves, finely chopped
- 2 tablespoons lemon juice
- 1 tablespoon garlic-infused olive oil
- Salt, to taste
- A pinch of black pepper

Nutrition (per serving):

35 calories | 2g fat | 3g carbs | 2g protein | 2g sugar

Prep. time: 10 min   **Total time:** 50 min   **Servings:** 2 cups

Directions:

1. In a medium bowl, combine the lactose-free Greek yogurt, finely chopped mint leaves, lemon juice, and garlic-infused olive oil.
2. Stir the mixture well until all the ingredients are thoroughly combined.
3. Add salt and black pepper to taste. Mix again to distribute the seasonings evenly.
4. To help the flavors combine, cover and chill the sauce for at least half an hour.
5. Serve the mint yogurt sauce chilled as a refreshing condiment for grilled meats, as a dip for vegetables, or drizzled over salads.

Vegan Alfredo Sauce

Ingredients:

- 1 cup raw cashews, soaked in water for 4 hours, then drained
- 1 cup unsweetened almond milk (or other low FODMAP nut milk)
- 2 tablespoons Nutrition (per serving):al yeast
- 2 tablespoons lemon juice
- 1 tablespoon garlic-infused olive oil
- 1/2 teaspoon salt
- 1/4 teaspoon black pepper
- 1/4 teaspoon ground nutmeg (optional)

Prep. time: 10 min   **Total time:** 25 min   **Servings:** 2 cups

Directions:

1. Blend the soaked and drained cashews, almond milk, Nutrition (per serving):al yeast, lemon juice, garlic-infused olive oil, salt, black pepper, and nutmeg if using.
2. Process on high until the mixture reaches a smooth and creamy consistency, about 2-3 minutes. If the sauce is too thick, add a little more almond milk until you reach your desired consistency.
3. Adjust the seasoning, adding extra salt, pepper, or lemon juice to suit your taste.
4. Transfer the sauce to a saucepan and warm it through over low heat, stirring occasionally to prevent sticking.
5. Serve the vegan Alfredo sauce over cooked low FODMAP pasta, steamed vegetables, or use it as a creamy base for other dishes.

Nutrition (per serving):

140 calories | 10g fat | 8g carbs | 5g protein | 2g sugar

Nut Butter

Prep. time: 10 min **Total time:** 20 min **Servings:** 16

Ingredients:

- 2 cups raw walnuts or macadamia nuts (or a mix of both, ensuring they're tolerated in your diet)
- 1/4 tsp salt (optional)
- 1 tbsp maple syrup (optional for a touch of sweetness)
- 1/4 tsp vanilla extract (optional)

Nutrition (per serving):

100 calories | 9g fat | 3g carbs | 2g protein | 1g sugar

Directions:

1. Preheat your oven to 350°F (175°C). Arrange the nuts in a single layer on a baking sheet.
2. Toast the nuts in the preheated oven for 8-10 minutes or until they are golden and fragrant. Watch them closely to prevent burning.
3. Take the nuts out of the oven and allow them to cool slightly.
4. Transfer the nuts to a food processor. Add salt, maple syrup, and vanilla extract if using.
5. Process the mixture on high speed, scraping down the sides as necessary, until the nuts break down into a creamy, smooth butter. This process can take several minutes, depending on the power of your food processor.
6. Once the desired consistency is reached, transfer the nut butter to a clean jar and seal tightly.
7. The nut butter can be stored in the refrigerator for up to 2 weeks. For a creamier texture, allow the nut butter to come to room temperature before serving.

Chapter 8: Drinks
Herbal Iced Tea

Ingredients:

- 4 cups water
- 4 herbal tea bags (such as peppermint, chamomile, or rooibos)
- 1/4 cup fresh mint leaves
- 2 tbsp honey (optional, adjust to taste)
- Lemon slices, for garnish

Nutrition (per serving):

15 calories | 0g fat | 4g carbs | 0g protein | 4g sugar

Prep. time: 5 min   **Total time:** 10 min   **Servings:** 4

Directions:

1. Bring the water to a boil in a kettle or saucepan.
2. Remove from heat, add the herbal tea bags and fresh mint leaves.
3. Give the tea five minutes or so to steep according to the tea package directions for strength preference.
4. Remove the tea bags and mint leaves, then stir in the honey until dissolved, if using.
5. Let the tea cool to room temperature, then refrigerate until chilled.
6. Serve the iced tea over ice, garnished with lemon slices.

Lemon Lime Soda

Ingredients:

- Juice of 2 lemons
- Juice of 2 limes
- 1/4 cup sugar (or to taste)
- 4 cups sparkling water
- Ice cubes
- Lemon and lime slices (for garnish)

Nutrition (per serving):

60 calories | 0g fat | 16g carbs | 0g protein | 15g sugar

Prep. time: 5 min   **Total time:** 5 min   **Servings:** 4

Directions:

1. In a small bowl, mix the lemon and lime juices and sugar until dissolved.
2. Divide the juice mixture among four glasses filled with ice.
3. Pour sparkling water into each glass, and mix gently.
4. Garnish with slices of lemon and lime.
5. Serve immediately for a refreshing, fizzy drink.

Peppermint Tea

Prep. time: 5 min   **Total time:** 10 min   **Servings:** 4

Ingredients:

- 4 cups water
- a handful of fresh peppermint leaves

Nutrition (per serving):

0 calories | 0g fat | 0g carbs | 0g protein | 0g sugar

Directions:

1. Bring water to a boil in a kettle or saucepan.
2. Once the water is boiling, remove it from the heat and add fresh peppermint leaves.
3. Let the tea steep for around 5 minutes.
4. Strain out the peppermint leaves.
5. Serve the tea hot or cold. Allow it to cool and then refrigerate to serve chilled.

Cucumber Mint Infused Water

Prep. time: 5 min   **Total time:** 5 min   **Servings:** 4

Ingredients:

- 1 medium cucumber, thinly sliced
- 10 fresh mint leaves
- 4 cups cold water
- Ice cubes (optional)

Nutrition (per serving):

0 calories | 0g fat | 0g carbs | 0g protein | 0g sugar

Directions:

1. Combine the sliced cucumber and mint leaves in a large pitcher.
2. Fill the pitcher with cold water.
3. Stir gently to mix the ingredients.
4. Place in the fridge for at least 1 hour or overnight to allow the flavors to infuse.
5. Serve the infused water over ice, if desired.

This cucumber mint-infused water is a wonderfully refreshing and hydrating drink, ideal for staying cool on hot days. It's simple to make and adds a subtle flavor, making drinking water more enjoyable.

Berry Lemonade

Prep. time: 10 min **Total time:** 10 min **Servings:** 4

Ingredients:
- 1/2 cup fresh blueberries
- 1/2 cup fresh strawberries, hulled and halved
- 3/4 cup fresh lemon juice from 4-5 lemons
- 1/3 cup sugar or to taste
- 4 cups cold water
- Ice cubes
- Lemon slices and additional berries for garnish

Nutrition (per serving):
90 calories | 0g fat | 23g carbs | 0.5g protein | 20g sugar

Directions:
1. In a blender, combine the strawberries, blueberries, and lemon juice. Blend until smooth.
2. Strain the berry mixture through a fine mesh sieve into a large pitcher, pressing to release as much liquid as possible. Discard the solids.
3. Add the sugar to the pitcher and mix until it fully dissolves.
4. Pour in the cold water and stir to combine.
5. Chill in the refrigerator or serve right away over ice, garnished with lemon slices and additional berries.

Ginger Turmeric Tea

Prep. time: 5 min **Total time:** 15 min **Servings:** 4

Ingredients:
- 4 cups water
- 2 inches fresh ginger root, peeled and sliced finely
- 2 inches fresh turmeric root, peeled and thinly sliced (or 1 tsp ground turmeric)
- 1 tbsp honey (optional, to taste)
- 1 lemon, juiced

Nutrition (per serving):
20 calories | 0g fat | 5g carbs | 0g protein | 4g sugar

Directions:
1. In a blender, combine the strawberries, blueberries, and lemon juice. Blend until smooth.
2. Strain the berry mixture through a fine mesh sieve into a large pitcher, pressing to release as much liquid as possible. Discard the solids.
3. Add the sugar to the pitcher and mix until it fully dissolves.
4. Pour in the cold water and stir to combine.
5. Chill in the refrigerator or serve right away over ice, garnished with lemon slices and additional berries.

Maple Cinnamon Latte

Prep. time: 5 min   **Total time:** 10 min   **Servings:** 2

Ingredients:

- 2 cups lactose-free milk or almond milk
- 2 tbsp maple syrup
- 1/2 tsp ground cinnamon
- 2 shots of espresso or 1/2 cup strong brewed coffee
- Whipped cream for topping (lactose-free if necessary)
- Additional cinnamon for sprinkling

Directions:

1. In a small saucepan, heat the lactose-free milk or almond milk over medium heat until it begins to simmer. Do not boil.
2. Add the ground cinnamon and maple syrup and stir.
3. Brew the coffee or espresso.
4. Divide the coffee or espresso between two mugs.
5. Pour the heated spiced milk into the mugs with the coffee.
6. Add whipped cream to the top of each mug and a sprinkle of additional cinnamon.
7. Serve immediately and enjoy your warm, comforting beverage.

Nutrition (per serving):

150 calories | 3g fat | 25g carbs | 5g protein | 18g sugar

Kiwi Strawberry Slush

Prep. time: 10 min   **Total time:** 10 min   **Servings:** 4

Ingredients:

- 2 ripe kiwis, peeled and quartered
- 1 cup fresh strawberries, hulled and halved
- 1 cup ice cubes
- 1/2 cup cold water
- 2 tbsp sugar (adjust to taste)
- 1 tbsp fresh lime juice

Directions:

1. In a blender, combine the kiwis, strawberries, ice cubes, cold water, sugar, and lime juice.
2. Blend at a high speed until the mixture is smooth and the ice is finely chopped.
3. Pour the slush into glasses and serve right away.

Nutrition (per serving):

70 calories | 0g fat | 18g carbs | 1g protein | 15g sugar

Golden Latte

Prep. time: 5 min   **Total time:** 10 min   **Servings:** 2

Ingredients:

- 2 cups lactose-free milk or almond milk
- 1 tsp ground turmeric
- 1/2 tsp ground cinnamon
- 1/4 tsp ground ginger
- Pinch of black pepper
- 1 tbsp honey or maple syrup (optional, to taste)
- 1/2 tsp vanilla extract

Nutrition (per serving):

120 calories | 5g fat | 15g carbs | 5g protein | 10g sugar

Directions:

1. In a small saucepan, combine the lactose-free milk or almond milk with the turmeric, cinnamon, ginger, and black pepper.
2. Stirring continuously, warm the mixture over medium heat until it is hot but not boiling.
3. Remove from heat and stir in the maple syrup or honey (if using) for more sweetness and vanilla extract.
4. Run the mixture through a strainer with fine mesh into two mugs to remove any large spices.
5. Serve warm, with an additional sprinkle of cinnamon on top for garnish if desired.

This warming Golden Latte, also known as turmeric latte, combines the anti-inflammatory benefits of turmeric with the comforting flavors of cinnamon and ginger, making it a soothing beverage ideal for relaxation or a gentle start to your day. Taste and adjust the spices and sweetness to match your preferences.

Chapter 9: 30-Day Meal Plan

Day 1:

- **Breakfast:** Low FODMAP Oatmeal with Maple Syrup and Walnuts
- **Lunch:** Quinoa Salad with Grilled Chicken and FODMAP-friendly Veggies
- **Dinner:** Baked Cod with Lemon and Herbs, served with Mashed Potatoes

Day 2:

- **Breakfast:** Berry Smoothie
- **Lunch:** Turkey Meatballs with a Side of Carrots
- **Dinner:** Low FODMAP Spaghetti Bolognese

Day 3:

- **Breakfast:** Quinoa Pancakes
- **Lunch:** Grilled Chicken Caesar Salad
- **Dinner:** Lemon Pepper Salmon with a Side of Rice

Day 4:

- **Breakfast:** Walnut and Seeds Granola with Lactose-free Milk
- **Lunch:** FODMAP-friendly Vegetable Stir-Fry with Tofu
- **Dinner:** Italian Meatloaf with Low FODMAP Vegetables

Day 5:

- **Breakfast:** Smoothie Bowl with Strawberries and Kiwi
- **Lunch:** Broccoli and Bacon Salad
- **Dinner:** Lemon Chicken with Herb Roasted Potatoes

Day 6:

- **Breakfast:** Rice Cakes with Lactose-Free Cream Cheese and Cucumber
- **Lunch:** Egg Salad with Dill
- **Dinner:** Pork Tenderloin with Oregano and Orange served with Polenta

Day 7:

- **Breakfast:** Chia Pudding with Coconut Milk and Raspberries
- **Lunch:** Turkey and Rice Soup
- **Dinner:** Grilled Mackerel with Herb Salad

Day 8:

- **Breakfast:** French Toast (made with gluten-free bread)
- **Lunch:** Zucchini Noodle Salad with Grilled Chicken
- **Dinner:** Beef and Fennel Casserole with Basmati Rice

Day 9:

- **Breakfast:** Scrambled Eggs with Spinach (use lactose-free milk)
- **Lunch:** Chicken and Orange Salad
- **Dinner:** Beef Stir-fry with Ginger and Bell Peppers (green only)

Day 10:

- **Breakfast:** Gluten-Free Cornflakes with Lactose-Free Milk
- **Lunch:** Golden Polenta Cakes with Spinach and Parmesan
- **Dinner:** Baked Trout with Dill and Lemon, served with Quinoa

Day 11:

- **Breakfast:** Blueberry Chia Overnight Oats
- **Lunch:** Miso Soup with Tofu and Greens
- **Dinner:** Lemon Herb Roasted Chicken, served with a side of FODMAP-friendly Ratatouille

Day 12:

- **Breakfast:** Strawberry Smoothie (use lactose-free milk)
- **Lunch:** Quinoa and Roasted Vegetable Salad with Pumpkin Seeds
- **Dinner:** Lemon Thyme Pork Tenderloin, served with Mashed Potatoes

Day 13:

- **Breakfast:** Mediterranean Vegetable Omelet
- **Lunch:** Minestrone Soup (omit onions and garlic)
- **Dinner:** Grilled Tilapia with Oregano and Olive Oil, served with Basmati Rice

Day 14:

- **Breakfast:** Low FODMAP Granola with Lactose-Free Yogurt
- **Lunch:** Chicken and Olive Pasta Salad (use gluten-free pasta)
- **Dinner:** Spiced Moroccan Chicken, served with Grilled Zucchini Ribbons

Day 15:

- **Breakfast:** Buckwheat Pancakes
- **Lunch:** Greek Salad with Feta (omit onions)
- **Dinner:** Lemon Pepper Salmon, served with Steamed Green Beans

Day 16:

- **Breakfast:** Omelet with Feta and Spinach
- **Lunch:** Seafood Paella
- **Dinner:** Slow-Cooked Beef with Carrots and Potatoes

Day 17:

- **Breakfast:** Sweet Potato and Walnuts Bowl
- **Lunch:** Rice Noodles with Grilled Chicken and Low FODMAP Veggies (like carrots and zucchini)
- **Dinner:** Maple Mustard Pork Chops with a side of Low FODMAP Coleslaw

Day 18:

- **Breakfast:** Italian Bruschetta (made with gluten-free bread)
- **Lunch:** Baked Falafel with a Low FODMAP Tzatziki Sauce
- **Dinner:** Herbed Turkey Burgers with a side of Baked Fries

Day 19:

- **Breakfast:** Chia Pudding with Coconut Milk and Strawberries
- **Lunch:** Stuffed Bell Peppers with Quinoa and Turkey (green only)
- **Dinner:** Baked Trout with Dill and Lemon, served with Rice

Day 20:

- **Breakfast:** Egg Bites with Ham
- **Lunch:** Lentil Soup with Carrots and Kale
- **Dinner:** Moroccan Spiced Lamb Ribs with Mint Sauce, served with Roasted FODMAP-friendly Veggies

Day 21:
- **Breakfast:** Turkey and Cheddar Breakfast Biscuits
- **Lunch:** Mini Caprese Salad
- **Dinner:** Baked Sea Bass with Fennel and Tomatoes

Day 22:
- **Breakfast:** Polenta with Feta
- **Lunch:** Lentil Soup (ensure lentils are rinsed well to reduce FODMAPs)
- **Dinner:** Grilled Cod with Lemon Butter Sauce and a side of Polenta

Day 23:
- **Breakfast:** Gluten-Free Pumpkin Bread
- **Lunch:** Turkey and Swiss Cheese Roll-ups with a side of Bell Peppers (green only)
- **Dinner:** Prawn Sti Fry

Day 24:
- **Breakfast:** Oatmeal with Maple Syrup and Chopped Walnuts
- **Lunch:** Spinach and Feta Quiche (gluten-free crust)
- **Dinner:** Beef and Broccoli Stir Fry (made with a gluten-free tamari sauce)

Day 25:
- **Breakfast:** Low FODMAP Muesli with Lactose-Free Milk
- **Lunch:** Greek Salad with Chicken (omit onions)
- **Dinner:** Fennel and Salmon Bake

Day 26:

- **Breakfast:** Scrambled Eggs with Chives and Lactose-Free Cheese
- **Lunch:** Chicken and Orange Salad
- **Dinner:** Rosemary Infused Roast Beef

Day 27:

- **Breakfast:** Baked Oatmeal Cups
- **Lunch:** Roasted Potato Salad
- **Dinner:** Roasted Chicken with Fennel and Potatoes

Day 28:

- **Breakfast:** Gluten-Free Porridge with Raisins and Cinnamon
- **Lunch:** Tuna Salad (with lactose-free mayo)
- **Dinner:** Maple Mustard Pork Chops, served with Sauteed Spinach

Day 29:

- **Breakfast:** French Toast (made with gluten-free bread)
- **Lunch:** Quinoa and Roasted Vegetable Salad
- **Dinner:** Grilled Shrimp with Garlic-Infused Olive Oil and a side of Greek

Day 30:

- **Breakfast:** Low FODMAP Smoothie with Lactose-Free Yogurt and Frozen Berries
- **Lunch:** Chicken and Rice Soup
- **Dinner:** Maple Glazed Turkey Meatballs with Mashed Potatoes

This plan covers a whole month with varied meals that adhere to low FODMAP guidelines, designed to be easy to prepare and delicious, helping to manage digestive comfort. Each recipe should be tailored to personal dietary needs and FODMAP tolerance levels.

Conclusion

As we reach the end of this culinary journey together in "The Essential Low FODMAP Diet Cookbook," I hope you feel empowered, informed, and inspired. Managing Irritable Bowel Syndrome (IBS) and other digestive disorders can often feel like an uphill battle, but with the right tools and knowledge, it is possible to live a life not dictated by your symptoms.

Throughout this book, we've explored over 130 easy and delicious recipes, each crafted to not only respect the principles of the Low FODMAP diet but also to bring joy and variety to your meals. From the inviting warmth of a nutritious soup to the simple joy of a freshly baked treat, these recipes ensure that everyone around your table can enjoy them, regardless of their digestive needs.

Moreover, the inclusion of a complete 30-day meal plan is intended to simplify your journey towards gut wellness. This plan serves as a roadmap, guiding you through breakfasts, lunches, dinners, and snacks while ensuring that you maintain a balanced intake of nutrients without feeling restricted or overwhelmed.

The goal of this cookbook was not just to ease your symptoms, but also to reintroduce a sense of delight and creativity into your cooking and eating habits. Food is one of life's greatest pleasures, and a dietary approach to managing health conditions shouldn't detract from that pleasure.

As you continue to use this cookbook, remember that each individual's response to different foods can vary. I encourage you to use the recipes and the meal plan as starting points. Experiment with flavors and ingredients within the Low FODMAP guidelines and tailor your diet to what feels best for your body. Your journey to gut wellness is deeply personal, and your diet can be just as unique.

Thank you for allowing me to be a part of your journey toward better health. Whether you're newly diagnosed with IBS, a long-time sufferer seeking relief, or a caretaker for someone with digestive issues, I hope this book becomes a resource you turn to often—not just for support. Keep striving for wellness, keep exploring new tastes, and remember: you have the power to transform your life, one meal at a time.

Here's to many more days of health, happiness, and hearty meals!

Appendix 1: Low FODMAP and High FODMAP Food Lists

Low FODMAP Foods

Vegetables: Alfalfa sprouts, bamboo shoots, bell peppers, bok choy, carrots, chives, cucumbers, eggplant, endive, ginger, green beans, kale, lettuce, olives, parsnips, potatoes, radishes, red bell peppers, scallions (green part only), spinach, squash (such as butternut and acorn), tomatoes, turnips, zucchini.

Fruits: Bananas (unripe), blueberries, cantaloupe, dragon fruit, grapes, kiwifruit, lemons, limes, mandarins, oranges, papaya, pineapple, raspberries, rhubarb, strawberries, tangerines.

Proteins: Beef, chicken, eggs, firm tofu, fish (such as cod, salmon, trout), lamb, pork, shellfish (such as shrimp, crab), tempeh, turkey.

Grains: Corn (including popcorn), oats, quinoa, rice, sourdough spelt bread, gluten-free breads and pastas, teff, millet, polenta.

Dairy and Dairy Alternatives: Almond milk, coconut milk, hemp milk, lactose-free milk, rice milk, soy milk (made with soy protein), cheddar cheese, feta cheese, mozzarella, parmesan, Swiss cheese, and other hard cheeses.

Nuts and Seeds: Almonds (small servings), brazil nuts, macadamia nuts, peanuts, pecans, pine nuts, pumpkin seeds, sesame seeds, sunflower seeds, walnuts.

Condiments and Sweeteners: Garlic-infused oil, ginger paste, maple syrup, mustard, soy sauce, wasabi, vinegar (except balsamic and apple cider).

Cheeses like cheddar, feta, mozzarella, parmesan, and Swiss are considered low FODMAP when consumed in small quantities, typically around 40 grams or 1.4 ounces. These cheeses are generally well tolerated because they contain lower lactose levels than softer cheeses.

High FODMAP Foods

Vegetables: Broccoli, artichokes, asparagus, Brussels sprouts, cabbage, cauliflower, fennel, garlic, leeks, mushrooms, onions, peas, shallots, snow peas, sugar snap peas, sweet corn, beetroot, celery, chicory leaves.

Fruits: Apples, apricots, avocado, blackberries, boysenberries, cherries, figs, mangoes, nectarines, peaches, pears, plums, prunes, watermelon, lychee, pomegranate, canned fruit in natural juice, dates.

Proteins: Legumes and pulses (beans, lentils, chickpeas, soybeans, baked beans, kidney beans, butter beans).

Grains: Barley, rye, wheat-based products (bread, pasta, cereals), couscous, semolina, amaranth, bulgur, kamut, spelt.

Dairy Products: Cow's milk, cream, custard, ice cream, soft cheeses (cottage cheese, ricotta, mascarpone), yogurt, sour cream, cream cheese.

Nuts and Seeds: Cashews, pistachios, hazelnuts, almonds (in large servings), mixed nuts.

Sweeteners: Agave nectar, fructose, honey, high-fructose corn syrup, isomalt, maltitol, mannitol, sorbitol, xylitol, molasses, coconut sugar.

Others: Chicory root, inulin, processed foods containing FODMAPs as additives, garlic and onion salts and powders, relishes and chutneys containing high FODMAP ingredients, soy sauce (in large amounts).

This list now includes a wider variety of high FODMAP foods, providing a more comprehensive reference for those needing to avoid or limit these in their diet.

Importance of Serving Size in FODMAP Levels

Understanding the importance of serving size is critical when following a low FODMAP diet, as the FODMAP content of food can vary significantly based on the amount consumed. Even foods typically considered high in FODMAPs can be suitable for a low FODMAP diet when eaten in smaller portions.

Examples of High FODMAP Foods Tolerable in Smaller Portions

- **Broccoli**: While the stalks are high in FODMAPs, the heads are much lower. A serving of 3/4 cup of chopped broccoli heads is considered low in FODMAPs.

- **Avocado**: Known for its high FODMAP content, a small serving of avocado (about 1/8 of a whole avocado) is low enough in FODMAPs to be tolerable for most people.

- **Sweet Corn**: Often avoided on a low FODMAP diet, sweet corn can be consumed in small amounts — about 1/2 cob — without exceeding low FODMAP limits.

- **Mushrooms**: While generally high in FODMAPs, certain types, like oyster mushrooms, can be low FODMAP at a serving size of 1 cup.

Properly managing portion sizes can significantly affect the success of a low FODMAP diet. By understanding which foods can be included in smaller amounts, individuals can enjoy a wider variety of foods while still adhering to a low FODMAP regimen. Using resources like the Monash University FODMAP Diet app ensures that individuals have access to reliable, research-based information to help make informed decisions about their diet.

This nuanced approach to portion control allows for a more flexible and manageable diet, potentially improving both physical comfort and quality of life for those with FODMAP sensitivities.

Appendix 2: Resource Recommendation

Websites

- **Monash University FODMAP Website**: The creators of the Low FODMAP diet, Monash University, offer extensive information, research updates, and practical guides on FODMAPs. Their website is a vital resource for scientific insights and expert advice.

- **The International Foundation for Gastrointestinal Disorders (IFFGD)**: A nonprofit organization that provides comprehensive information on GI disorders, including resources specifically for those following a Low FODMAP diet.

- **FODMAP Everyday:** A website dedicated to helping those on the Low FODMAP diet live easier, better, and more delicious lives through a wealth of recipes, shopping guides, and meal planning tips.

Mobile Apps

- **Monash University FODMAP Diet App:** Created by the team at Monash University, this app is a vital resource for anyone following a Low FODMAP diet. It offers comprehensive details regarding the FODMAP content of hundreds of foods, updated with the latest research findings, and helps users identify which parts of certain foods are lower in FODMAPs. The app includes a comprehensive guide to food portion sizes, FODMAP content, and a food diary feature to track your meals and symptoms.

    Available on iOS and Android.

- **FODMAP Helper - Diet Companion:** This app helps identify foods that are safe to eat and those you should stay away from. It includes a detailed list of Low and High FODMAP foods and provides personal food ratings based on your tolerances.

    Available on iOS and Android.

Appendix 3: Measurement Conversions

Measurement Type	Imperial	Metric
Volume	1 teaspoon	5 milliliters
	1 tablespoon	15 milliliters
	1 fluid ounce	30 milliliters
	1 cup	240 milliliters
	1 pint (2 cups)	470 milliliters
	1 quart (4 cups)	950 milliliters
	1 gallon (16 cups)	3.8 liters
Weight	1 ounce	28 grams
	1 pound (16 oz)	454 grams
Temperature	32°F	0°C (freezing point of water)
	212°F	100°C (boiling point of water)
	250°F	120°C
	275°F	135°C
	300°F	150°C
	325°F	160°C
	350°F	175°C
	375°F	190°C
	400°F	200°C
	425°F	220°C
	450°F	230°C

Cooking on the Low FODMAP diet requires precision, not just in selecting ingredients but also in measuring them. This appendix provides conversion tables for common measurements used in cooking and baking, facilitating easy and accurate recipe adjustments.

Using this appendix, you can confidently adjust recipes from different parts of the world to fit your diet and kitchen equipment. Accurate measurement is key to maintaining a balanced Low FODMAP diet and achieving the desired outcomes for your recipes.

Printed in Great Britain
by Amazon